SISTERS OF
MOKAMA

SISTERS OF
MOKAMA

The Pioneering Women
Who Brought Hope and
Healing to India

Jyoti Thottam

VIKING

VIKING

An imprint of Penguin Random House LLC
penguinrandomhouse.com

LIBRARY OF CONGRESS CATALOGING-IN-PUBLICATION DATA

Names: Thottam, Jyoti, author.
Title: Sisters of Mokama : the pioneering women who brought hope and
healing to India / Jyoti Thottam.
Description: New York : Viking, [2022] | Includes bibliographical references.
Identifiers: LCCN 2021039059 (print) | LCCN 2021039060 (ebook) |
ISBN 9780525522355 (hardcover) | ISBN 9780525522362 (ebook)
Subjects: LCSH: Women in medicine—India. | Women—Health and hygiene—India. |
Nurses—History—Biography. | Nuns—India—Biography.
Classification: LCC R692 .T47 2022 (print) | LCC R692 (ebook) |
DDC 610.82—dc23/eng/20211124
LC record available at https://lccn.loc.gov/2021039059
LC ebook record available at https://lccn.loc.gov/2021039060

Printed in the United States of America
1   3   5   7   9   10   8   6   4   2
CJKB

Set in Sabon MT Std
Designed by Cassandra Garruzzo Mueller

To my parents,
George and Elsamma Thottam

Contents

Introduction

In my favorite photograph of my parents, they are newlyweds visiting the Taj Mahal, in 1971. They are posing on the long, graceful stone pathway, with the curves of the monument far behind them, decades before India had become pockmarked with construction sites, so the view of the Taj is absolutely clear. The spouts for the fountains in the reflecting pool are idle, but the water shimmers. There are no hawkers, no elaborate system of security checkpoints or shoe removal visible at the stone pedestal in the distance. The only objects between my parents and the monument are a line of trees, manicured into tall evergreen pillars.

Young and serious, they had decided to visit the Taj Mahal during the cool late winter, and the photograph hints at their life before I was born. They stand soberly in their best clothes: my father in a three-button suit and tightly knotted skinny tie, and my mother with the peacock-blue sari that was given to her as a ceremonial gift during their wedding draped modestly around her shoulders.

My parents had been living in New Delhi for years by then. My father moved there in 1961; my mother a few years later. The city, India's capital, was more than a thousand miles away from the tiny villages in the south where they were born. It was farther than most people in India at that time would travel in a lifetime. My father had come north to work for a civil engineering firm that built some of independent India's first big roads, dams, and skyscrapers. He still tells the story of the cold, wet weeks he spent in the Himalayas, supervising the construction of a bridge during India's 1962 war with China.

Most men of his generation went home to find an appropriate wife, but my parents fell in love in the big city. They met in Delhi in 1969, when my mother was twenty-two, living in a hostel and working as a nurse. She had arrived in the city after seven years studying nursing in a small town in Bihar, at a school run by American nuns. He saw her at church, and then again at the market, and fell in love at first sight. He courted her modestly—a meal at the home of his elder brother and sister-in-law, an ice cream at Kwality, and eventually the movies, once she trusted him enough to ride on the back of his Vespa scooter.

If you ask her about it now, she repeats this story as if it were the most ordinary thing in the world. Of course, there was much more to it. My mother was born in 1946, a year before Partition, when Britain's vast colonial empire on the subcontinent was split into two countries, India and Pakistan. Independence had been decades in the making, but except for the principle that Pakistan would be majority Muslim and India mostly Hindu, little was clear about what these new nations would be. Would they welcome or tolerate religious minorities? Could they bind together people who spoke dozens of different languages? Would they ever give redress to the Indigenous people who had been displaced from their land, or those forced to work on it under the oppressions of caste? Without any answers to those questions, hundreds of millions of people had to choose sides and stake their claim to a place, somewhere. This quest sent millions on the move, and unleashed waves of violence in the months before and after Partition, and repercussions for years afterward.

My mother was part of a generation of women who inherited all the burdens of the past and yet found the will and the means to reject them. She pursued her own career, made her own money, and chose her own husband. The demure bride in the photograph was also a woman who made her way into the world and never looked back.

She was a schoolgirl, just fifteen years old, when she left her home at the southern tip of India, in the state of Kerala, and traveled to Bihar, a place known even then as the poorest and most violent in India. The train took her to a small market town called Mokama,* built up around a railroad junction at a bend in the river Ganges. It was little more than a few shops serving the railway workers and big landowners. And yet, a few minutes walk from the railway station, there was a grand Catholic church, a hospital, and a nursing school run by a handful of nuns from Kentucky.

My mother remembers the sisters with a mix of emotions: they were strict and enforced their rules mercilessly, they were tall and pale, they spoke with incomprehensible accents, they were uncompromising in their standards, they taught her everything she knows about nursing, they looked after her for years, they indulged her, they changed her life.

Beyond the limits of these family stories, there was so much more I wanted to know. How did she manage to travel so far, at such a young age, when few women dared to leave their homes without the protection of a man? Why Bihar? And why did these nuns choose to start a hospital in Mokama, a town so small it didn't appear on most

---

* The town was usually spelled "Mokameh" at the time, but I have used the contemporary spelling here and elsewhere. For most other place names, including Bombay and Calcutta, I have used the spellings most common at the time.

maps of India? Why did they leave Kentucky and come to this particular corner of India, just months after Partition, to a place that had been scarred by violence between Hindus and Muslims? And why did they fill that hospital with teenage nurses from the other end of the country? Did they have any idea how radical their work would be? They started a hospital and school run almost entirely by women, and they insisted on giving the highest possible standard of care to everyone who walked through the doors, regardless of caste or religion.

These were questions I would have to answer myself, as a journalist, over the course of years of research. I made my first trip to Mokama in 1998, contacting the sisters through what was still the most reliable means of communication: the mail. I sent them a letter asking if I might visit, and then another a few weeks later to let them know which train I planned to take. I was traveling around India at the time, and tried repeatedly to reach them by phone to confirm that they would be able to meet me at the station.

I was reluctant to travel there alone; Bihar was a dangerous place, the site of a gang war between rival castes. I was unable to reach them by phone, so eventually I took a deep breath, bought my train ticket, sent them a telegram with the name of the train and its arrival time, and hoped for the best. It was an overnight train from Delhi, going east across Uttar Pradesh. I knew exactly when we had crossed the state line into Bihar; it was the moment the ticketless travelers began jumping into the compartments. As we got closer, the train slowed in the middle of the night and came to a stop. There was a body on the tracks. I couldn't determine who had been killed or how. But I resolved to myself that if there was no one to meet me when I reached Mokama, I would simply remain at the station and take the next train back to Delhi. I arrived at Mokama Junction in the bright morning sun, and two of the sisters were there waiting for me. The delay turned out to have been fortuitous. My telegram had arrived just before the train, so if it had come on time, they would have missed it.

I spent a few days in Mokama on that trip. Mostly, I just wanted to see the place that had loomed so large in my imagination and in the story of my family. The town was surrounded by lush, green farmland, but the sisters' description of life there was terrifying. A woman who studied there in the 1970s and '80s remembered lying awake at night listening for the beating of horses' hooves—the sound of violence on its way. The caste wars that began during Partition had continued and multiplied, as caste-based militias, sometimes including men on horseback, splintered into rival factions. Nazareth Hospital had become the place where victims of violent crime—gunshots, bomb blasts, knife attacks—came to be treated, no questions asked. It was the only place that had no allegiance to either side.

More than a decade later, I traveled to Bihar again. I was in the middle of a four-year posting as *Time* magazine's bureau chief in New Delhi, and the state was then in the middle of an unlikely resurgence. Say "Bihar" to almost anyone in India, and the word evokes a predictable response: Why would you go there? It's so miserable, so poor, so corrupt, so violent. It is, for India, the equivalent of the Mississippi delta or the favelas of Rio de Janeiro. But a new chief minister had recently taken over leadership of the state, and I saw during several trips to Bihar that he seemed to be making some progress in easing the violence and hopelessness.

The more I learned about Bihar, the more I realized how remarkable the story of Nazareth Hospital really was—for women like my mother who studied there in the 1960s, and also for the American women who had started it in 1947. I was desperate to learn more about them. So I contacted the order, the Sisters of Charity of Nazareth, through its headquarters in Kentucky, and asked if it might be possible to talk to any of the original six American nuns who had started the hospital. The youngest was still alive: Ann Roberta Powers, born Roberta Powers in Cloverport, Kentucky.

"That's my name, it's been that way since 1924," she said by way of introduction. We met in the cool, spacious parlor of a convent in Gaya, another city in Bihar, where Ann Roberta had come to spend her last years. She was the youngest and the last surviving "pioneer sister," as her order called those who founded the mission in Mokama in 1947. When I met her she was eighty-six, a tiny, plump woman in a gauzy, flowered sari. For two hours she described in vivid detail her childhood in Cloverport: the Catholic schools where she and her sisters earned their keep as working boarders, and the traveling missionary whose stories inspired her to seek a glimpse of the world outside Kentucky.

Ann Roberta was only twenty-two when she left America in 1947—she had not even taken her final vows, the last step in making a lifetime commitment to religious life—and the two-month journey from Kentucky to India, by ship and cross-country train, was the adventure of a lifetime. She recited the dates and details as if she had stepped off the ship only days earlier. She told me about the first months of setting up the hospital—scrounging for supplies, improvising beds and bandages, planting a garden, and learning to bargain for vegetables in Hindi with merchants in the bazaar. I asked her what kind of patients they would get in those early days, and she immediately recalled the orphans. This was in the first years after the traumatic Partition that split the subcontinent into India and Pakistan. Twelve million people left their homes, fleeing violence or taking a chance on a new life on the other side of the newly drawn borders, and families were scattered in every direction.

She told me about one little girl who was brought to the hospital from the train station at Mokama by the railway police. She was still a toddler, well fed and beautiful. That in itself was unusual—most of the orphans who landed at Nazareth Hospital arrived malnourished and sick. But this girl had been traveling with her mother on a train from Delhi to Calcutta. About halfway through the journey, as the train halted at a station in the middle of the night, the mother told the other people in the compartment that she wanted to get some more milk for her child. Would they mind keeping an eye on her while she slept?

The mother never came back. The other passengers thought she must have boarded in a different car and would walk back to her berth, but when the train reached the next station, Mokama, she still had not returned.

They called the railway police, who brought the abandoned child to the convent. The nuns carried her inside to examine her. She was lethargic, perhaps drugged, but otherwise healthy. She wore a diaper— a soft, store-bought one, a luxury at the time. The nuns began to undress her to put her to bed and discovered that she was wearing six frilly dresses, one on top of the other. They must have been all the clothing she owned in the world.

Ann Roberta paused for a moment over that detail, stunning in its tenderness and cruelty. It was St. Bernard's Day, so they called her Marie Bernadette.

That was the moment I felt that there was more to the story of Nazareth Hospital than I had imagined. It was built out of the ashes of Partition, a place where those who had escaped or endured the ruptures of home and community would learn to look at this new and brutal world for what it was. When you could no longer count on anyone to protect you, where would you go? What would you do?

Who would you be? What kind of place was India in 1947, where a woman might lovingly prepare her own child to be abandoned?

There were thousands of such children in India at the time, orphans whose parents had been killed in the months of violence and others who were left behind in the great rush of people fleeing from one place to another. This girl didn't look like a refugee. She could have been the child of a marriage between a Hindu and a Muslim. During Partition, the lines between communities hardened. Parents and children, husbands and wives were sometimes forced to choose between one country and the other. She could have been the product of rape. There were thousands of women, on both sides of the border, who suffered sexual violence, and it took many months for the governments of India and Pakistan to decide the fate of their children. There were also thousands of husbands who went off to fight or to find their fortunes on the other side of the Partition line, and it was not uncommon for months to pass without their sending word back to their wives. Had the child's mother been one of those wives, who took a lover to fill the silence? Or perhaps she had simply decided to seize that moment, when the whole world was in chaos, to choose a different life for herself—another city, another name, another destiny, one that she would choose for herself.

In many ways, all the women of Nazareth—the sisters like Ann Roberta, who left their homes in Kentucky to go to India, and the young women like my mother, who left their villages to study nursing—were animated by the same impulse. The years after World War II in the United States and the years after Partition in India were, in one important way, the same: they were years of tumult and trauma, when those whose lives had been constrained by an old order found themselves suddenly free when that order was destroyed. Pain and loss were everywhere for the women of that time, but what looked like a vacuum was, for some women, an opening, a chance to create for themselves lives that would never have been possible otherwise.

Five years after my interview with Ann Roberta, in July 2016, I walked inside the motherhouse of the Sisters of Charity of Nazareth in Nelson County, Kentucky. It was a hot day, but the wide green lawns were shaded by dogwoods and redbuds. I passed the formal sitting rooms—where sisters in training had once approached visitors with the slow, dignified walk they had been taught—on the way to the archives. After months of gentle prodding, the leadership of the order had agreed to give me access to the records of the sisters' time in India.

Ann Roberta had died the year before. Her file in the archives was thick, filled with decades' worth of photographs and mementos. At the front of the file was a carefully filled-out card detailing the names of her parents, her siblings, her name when she entered the convent, the name she took with her vows, and the particulars of every mission to which she had been assigned during more than sixty years in the order.

I wore white cotton gloves to handle the fragile documents, and my hands trembled as I picked up Ann Roberta's passport. It was issued on July 18, 1947, No. 17363, and arrived at the British consulate in Chicago on July 30, 1947. Independence for India and Pakistan was two weeks away, so the British consulate still had the authority to approve her travel to India. And so, in one of his last acts as representative of the British Raj, the consular official granted her permission for a "Single Journey Authorized by the Government of India," writing the words in a flourish of black ink above a green eight-shilling stamp. It was valid for six months, for a single journey.

The pages of the passport are otherwise empty. Ann Roberta had

never ventured more than a few hundred miles from her home in Cloverport, Kentucky. I turned the pages to find her passport picture. She
smiled so widely with anticipation that her cheeks nearly touched the
sides of her starched cotton cap. Soon after it was taken, she visited
her family back in Cloverport to say her last goodbyes. The superiors had warned her that she would probably never see her family
again, but her face in this photo shows no trace of nervousness or
hesitation.

I spent months reading through the mission logs of the order, documents from the archives of the Archdiocese of Patna, as well as hundreds of letters that the sisters wrote home to their families during
their years in India, which revealed more about what motivated Ann
Roberta and the other sisters to make that leap. They were part of a
generation of women from Kentucky who grew up during the Depression and came of age during World War II, after which they
looked at the ashes of a broken world and saw that they could make
something new. In their letters, they rarely mentioned converting
souls to Christianity, although their faith permeated every part of
their lives. They had given themselves to the Church, but they knew,
too, that they had been given something in return: a chance to live out
a great adventure thousands of miles from home. They were, of
course, women who had dedicated their lives to the missionary goals
of the Catholic Church, and their very presence in India was met with
no small amount of hostility. But they were motivated by more than
simply religious fervor. They were American women in the postwar
era. They had chosen to be there, to rebuild a corner of India and to
create for themselves a new role as women in the Church.

When they arrived at the end of 1947, India was a devastated
country, enduring violence, dislocation, and food shortages on a mass
scale. By the end of 1948, two of India's cities, Delhi and Bombay, had

each absorbed more than 500,000 refugees. Calcutta absorbed 400,000. About 12,500 women who had been abducted, raped, and sometimes forced into marriages were returned, not always at their request, to families in India that may have rejected them. The country, which had been forced under the imperial war production policies to supply millions of tons of wheat and rice for British forces, was depleted. It could no longer produce enough for its own population. More than 20 million Indians lived under direct rationing, entitled to only ten ounces of grain a day.

Adding to the collective trauma, India lost Mohandas K. Gandhi, the Mahatma or "great soul," to an assassin's bullet in January 1948. It was a shock that came less than six months after Partition, marking another rupture for a country that had looked to Gandhi for much more than political leadership. He was the moral force behind the independence movement, and in the void he left behind the rest of India's political leaders had to articulate what India might be.

They gathered soon after the assassination in the "Constituent Assembly," a series of public meetings attended by representatives of nearly every community in India, to debate the principles and ideas that would animate the new nation's constitution. It was an extraordinary moment, similar to the constitutional conventions in which America's founding fathers wrote its Constitution, but this one was conducted in full public view, with each day's proceedings and eloquent speeches followed closely in the Indian press. The assembly embraced a vision of India that would not be defined by one saintly man or a return to some mythical ancient past. Jaipal Singh, an Oxford-educated civil servant who had captained the Indian field hockey team to a gold medal in the 1928 Olympics, represented the tribals of South Bihar, perhaps the poorest and most completely dispossessed communities in India. In his speech to the assembly, Singh offered a

version of India's history in which the Indigenous people of India considered everyone else—the Hindus and Mughals and the rest—to be
latecomers and asserted that the injustices suffered by Bihar's tribals
would finally be addressed. "We are now going to start a new chapter, a new chapter of independent India where there is equality of
opportunity, where no one is neglected."

The idealism embodied by the gathering feels breathtaking and
heartbreaking, given how far from those ideals India had fallen decades later. But it was a moment of crystalline hope. By 1948, nearly
all the remaining British civil servants had gone. That left an opening
for Americans, like the sisters in Mokama, who had come to India by
happenstance or ideology or folly. Albert Mayer, an American architect who worked in India in the early years of independence, described
"the tingling atmosphere of plans and expectation and uncertainty"
in India at the time. "What it adds up to is being present at the birth
of a nation."

Through various accidents of fate and history, the sisters from
Kentucky found common cause with Indian women like my mother.
She, too, was far from home, stepping into a life radically different
from the one she was born to. The young women who were trained at
Nazareth Hospital—some as nurses, some as sisters, and some in
both vocations—had desires that, in another era, could never have
been fulfilled.

The first years after Partition cast a harsh light. The country was
free from British rule, but this newly independent nation could not
fulfill the basic needs, let alone the hopes and ambitions, of most
of its people. That would require new institutions, new ideas, and
people—men and women—who were willing to take a chance on
building them.

The women whose stories fill these pages would never describe themselves as extraordinary. Their lives and choices helped shape the future of two nations, but what happened to them is fading from memory. For decades, the history of modern India seemed to end at Partition, and the final convulsions of a dying empire. Since then, scholars have begun to look more closely at Partition itself and the two decades after it, through oral histories and reconstructions of that personal and political trauma, and much of that history is still left to be explored.

I have tried to contribute to that work by looking at the first twenty years of independent India through the eyes of the women of Nazareth Hospital. I spoke to them in person whenever possible, and I spent hours on the phone interviewing them and their relatives. I made several visits to Mokama and the surrounding area, and I spent months immersing myself in the world of Nazareth Hospital.

What I found was a country in the process of becoming the nation as it's known today. Many observers of modern India date the beginning of the "new India"—the India of computer engineers and ambitious middle-class strivers—to the economic reforms of 1991. But I would argue that to understand contemporary India, one has to go back much further, to the restless young people of the 1950s and '60s.

There is a hint of this even in that photograph of my parents. When I look closely, I can see another couple in the image walking toward them, about halfway down the path. They are striding, not posed, and it is not entirely clear if they are married. The distance between them seems so casual; maybe they're friends or classmates or lovers. The woman is smiling, her hair is tied loosely behind her, and with her sari she wears high heels and a sleeveless blouse—the height of fashion at the time. The man is wearing a sweater and ill-fitting pants as he takes a drag from a cigarette with one hand and dangles a camera from a cord with the other. There is something so daring about that other couple—the bare arms, the cigarette. They remain unknown to me, but I think of them as part of my parents' story in India, when so much was new and everything seemed possible.

Although this is not intended as a memoir or family history, I am there, too, in that photograph, in the gentle swell of my mother's belly. This book is my effort to reclaim that history, for myself and for all the other children of Nazareth.

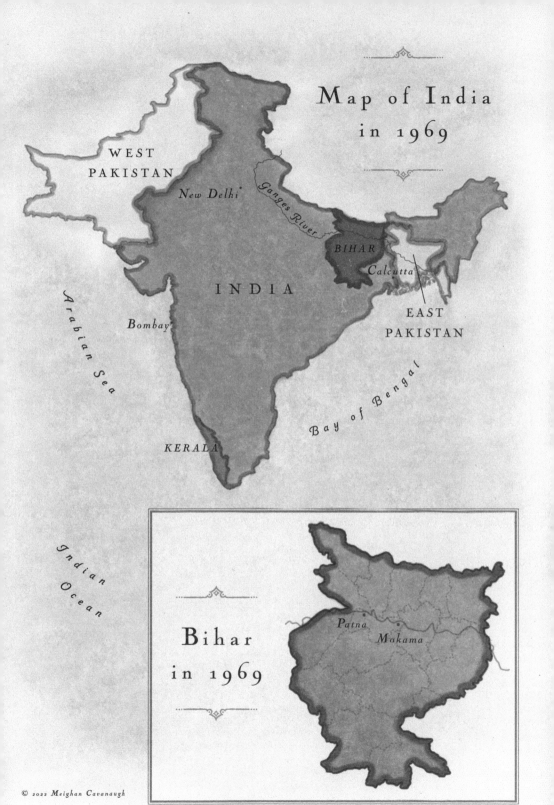

Map of India
in 1969

WEST
PAKISTAN

New Delhi

Ganges River

BIHAR

Calcutta

EAST
PAKISTAN

INDIA

Arabian Sea

Bombay

Bay of Bengal

KERALA

Indian
Ocean

Bihar
in 1969

Patna   Makama

© 2022 Meighan Cavanaugh

World War II hurled us into the twentieth century. . . . I began dreaming of a rootless way of life, one that would knock me loose from the rock-solid homestead and catapult me into the fluid, musical motions of faraway cities.

BOBBIE ANN MASON, *CLEAR SPRINGS*

ONE

The End of a Great War

On the evening of August 14, 1945, news of the Japanese emperor's surrender reached Nazareth, Kentucky. The chimes from the stone chapel next to the convent began to sound, and Ann Sebastian Sullivan, mother superior of the Sisters of Charity of Nazareth, listened as the ringing pierced the air, tumbling over the rolling green hills to join the church bells in nearby Bardstown, three and a half miles to the south.

Ann Sebastian moved her stately frame through the empty halls of the convent like a battleship, her black wool habit gliding over the polished wood floors. The rest of the nuns made their way to the chapel, gathering behind their superior as she bent over her prayer book, the edges curled and worn with use. They came to give thanks; the war was over.

Forty miles to the north, in Louisville, the news shook the city "like an erupting volcano." It started at about six in the evening, when an announcer climbed to the stage of the Scoop News Theatre, a vaudeville house at Walnut Street and Fourth Street. The crowds spilled outside, spreading the good news, and the factory whistles, automobile horns, and police sirens roused the city to life. Drivers heading down Fourth Street leaned on their horns in jubilation. Soon, the cars were immobilized, surrounded by people pouring into the streets.

A giddy spirit moved through the waves of revelers. A girl swaggered down the sidewalk in nothing but a pink bathing suit. A man in red-striped pajamas led an improvised marching band on dishpans and toy horns. Another shuffled down Fourth Street in an ill-considered tribute to the Pacific theater—a grass skirt, beads, and headdress. There were kisses bestowed on just about anyone in uniform. The bars shut early, so groups of soldiers clustered on the curb at Lincoln Park, passing around bottles of whiskey to toast their good fortune. Over at Churchill Downs, a Gershwin concert was interrupted only briefly by word of the surrender. The genteel crowd listened, as planned, to two soldiers—an opera singer and a pianist before their deployment—play the old favorites with the Louisville Philharmonic.

The newspapers had prepared Kentucky for this moment of release and celebration. The day before, *The Courier-Journal* tallied the cost to America, in blood and treasure, of nearly four years of conflict: almost $300 billion and more than a million casualties, including 250,000 dead.

Louisville was proud of the big role it had played in the war, given its small size. The military camps at nearby Fort Knox and Bowman Field housed more than 60,000 soldiers, and many of them passed through the USO headquarters downtown. The city was a crucial wartime production hub, too. Soon after Pearl Harbor, the War Department called Mayor Wilson Wyatt and told him to post extra guards near the Ohio River bridges and war plants in case of another sneak attack. There was a powder plant in nearby Charlestown, across the Ohio River; a chemical plant in Rubbertown; a naval ordnance plant; and the Ohio River shipyards. The Curtiss-Wright aircraft plant produced the C-76 emergency aircraft, and Louisville's Ford Motor Assembly Plant produced more than 93,000 of the 500,000 military jeeps that eventually entered service.

Wyatt was a New Dealer, a solid ally of Roosevelt, and he turned Louisville into a clearinghouse for civilian volunteers from all over the state. Kentucky's population of 3 million included more than 170,000 people working in war plants—60,000 of them women. There were 50,000 volunteers in Louisville alone. Even high school students had the chance to train at the Curtiss-Wright plant instead of attending class, if they kept their grades up, and the Ford dealership on Southwest Parkway turned its showroom into a display of army trucks.

But few volunteers generated as much local pride as the women of the airborne nursing service. Women, of course, had long assumed that caretaking role in wartime, but with this conflict, the first to be won from the air, nurses ventured into new and difficult territory. They trained at the air base at Bowman Field in sidearms, battlefield medicine, and camouflage, skills they would need when they encountered enemy soldiers while retrieving wounded men from forward positions.

The need for nurses was intense. Even before America entered the war, a census revealed a severe shortage. In 1940, only one hundred thousand nurses were qualified to serve in the military. At a gathering of nursing associations at the Army Nurse Corps headquarters in Washington, Mary Beard of the Red Cross Nursing Service warned, "I have no words to tell you how serious I believe this is going to be." Roosevelt called for a draft of nurses, and the federal government allocated $1.25 million for nursing education, although it would be years before those women would be ready to serve. Just before the

United States entered the fight, more than four thousand Red Cross nurses were transferred from reserve to active duty.

So it was all the more remarkable that Mother Ann Sebastian, whose order included more than 1,300 trained nurses and teachers, had refused to join the war effort overseas. On September 21, 1942, she wrote a letter to Dorothy Eveslage, secretary of the Lexington chapter of the American Red Cross, carefully choosing the words to explain herself: "We regret that shortage of personnel, together with pressure of work in our hospitals, prevents placing our sister nurses at the Government's disposal for the duration except for an emergency." The order was already running schools teaching more than twenty thousand students in Kentucky, and the Sisters of Charity were the primary nursing staff for four hospitals in three states, with two more planned to open. Unless there was an epidemic or emergency in the United States, Ann Sebastian wrote, she could not send her nurses into the fight. "We feel, however, that to operate our hospitals during this period is rendering service in complete accord with the wishes of our President."

The decision was baffling to the young nurses of the Sisters of Charity of Nazareth, who were ready to volunteer. Nearly all of them had brothers in the military, and they had watched the lay people they worked with answer the call. Just a year earlier, in July 1941, Rose Fitzgerald, a lay nurse who had helped the sisters run a clinic for African Americans in Birmingham, Alabama, was called up to active service. On the grounds of the convent in Nazareth, ninety-three-year-old Monroe Smith, who had once been enslaved on a farm in Nelson County and later, after winning his freedom, worked as a gardener on the convent grounds, took up additional work, raking leaves and burning trash to fill in for the men who had been called up. In Louisville, the sisters ran a day care center, making it possible for

mothers to start working in the defense plants. The sisters who were
trained as nurses were not permitted to use their valuable nursing
skills to help with the war effort, but the nursing journals they read
were filled with the exploits of brave nurses overseas. A nurse from
Scranton, Pennsylvania, served on the first army transport ship to arrive at Pearl Harbor after it was attacked, and army nurses were the
first American women to enter southern France with the invasion
forces after D-Day. But the nurses from the Sisters of Charity remained at home.

A century earlier, when Kentucky was still a frontier, the Sisters of
Charity had been among the heroines of these stories. During the
Spanish-American War, the sisters went to Chattanooga to care for
soldiers who had contracted pneumonia on the long journey to the
Caribbean. During the Civil War, the nuns from Nazareth treated
both Confederate and Union troops. One of them, Sister Mary Lucy
Dosh, died of an infection on the battlefield and was given a full military burial, with honor guards in blue and gray. Abraham Lincoln
himself had taken notice. On January 17, 1865, as General William
Sherman rested his rampaging troops in Savannah, Lincoln received
an urgent request from a Kentucky senator, Lazarus Powell. Union
troops had taken over several buildings belonging to the Sisters of
Charity, and Powell went to Lincoln to complain in person. Powell
was no favorite of Lincoln's—two weeks later, the senator would vote
against the Thirteenth Amendment—but he left the meeting with a
handwritten decree from the president: "Let no depredation be committed upon the property or possessions of the 'Sisters of Charity' at
Nazareth Academy, near Bardstown, Kentucky."

The early history of the order is inseparable from that of Kentucky.

The earliest Catholics in Kentucky were a league of sixty families who left Maryland and settled on Pottinger's Creek in Nelson County in 1785. The land was poor, so another group settled near the headwaters of the Salt River in Bardstown, where they built a cluster of log houses and, eventually, a church. One settler donated land and a house nearby in Nazareth that would serve as a residence for priests and nuns—a Catholic society can't sustain itself without Catholic schools run by Catholic women—and in 1813, the first Sisters of Charity took their vows.

Soon, this young Catholic community began to attract women with vocations, and a willingness to endure the hardships of life on the frontier, from the more established Catholic enclaves on the East Coast. At the time, that's what it meant to be an American Catholic missionary: to go west to serve the scattered Catholic population on the other side of the Allegheny Mountains.

Ann Sebastian Sullivan was among them. The daughter of an immigrant from County Kerry, she was born Catherine Sullivan in 1883 and came to Kentucky in 1905. Trained as a bookkeeper, she left her home in the large and established Irish Catholic community of Baltimore to follow her religious vocation.

When Ann Sebastian arrived in Nazareth, she began training as a teacher. Over the next two decades, she taught in Catholic schools in Ohio, Maryland, Tennessee, and Kentucky, eventually becoming the supervisor of all the Catholic schools in Louisville. By 1930, she was the "first councillor" to the mother superior, and six years later was elected superior of more than a thousand nuns.

By that point, Kentucky was no longer a frontier. The land was all but spent, and subsistence farming was becoming impossible. Some family farms survived the Depression by selling tobacco or timber, but that didn't last. Machines were replacing human and animal labor in the fields, so farmers left for the factories of Michigan, Illinois, Indiana, and Ohio. The remaining wealth of the state was sequestered in Louisville's commerce and Lexington's bluegrass estates.

As the frontier faded, the balance of power shifted between two competing ideals of white womanhood: the "competence and resourcefulness" of frontier women and the "useless and decorative" women of the cities. The bold, forthright style of the pioneers held sway in early Kentucky, when the state was not even a state, just mountains, rugged hills, and buffalo traces. Although its ideals persisted in imagination, actual frontier life vanished within a couple of decades. As plantations and then the steamboat trade along the Ohio River brought wealth to the state, other ideals of womanhood began to take hold—embodied in the genteel matrons of plantation Lexington and the cosmopolitan, ambitious aristocrats of Louisville.

By the 1820s, the change was noticeable. In her memoir, Mary Austin Holley, wife of the president of Transylvania University, the oldest in Kentucky, wrote that the log cabins had been replaced by handsome brick houses. "Gone too were frontier simplicity and egalitarianism." Women were no longer valued for their strength and skills—which were vital to the project of settling Indigenous land. Instead, they became living evidence of a family's financial success. Daughters were sheltered in their houses, educated in fashionable schools, and separated from the rest of urban life. Holley "preferred the more forthright manners of the early Republic in which she had been raised," but it had disappeared in a generation. Her married daughter, she noticed, had adopted the manners of the "new reticence."

Well into the twentieth century, a strict sense of propriety encircled Kentucky's women. The trousseau for a well-to-do Louisville bride included not just nightgowns, handmade lingerie, a going-away suit, white riding breeches, and a hunting jacket for fox hunts, but also "monogrammed satin panels she would use to cover her underwear when she left it on hotel room chairs."

Catholic girls' schools reinforced and, in some cases, taught these norms of modesty and propriety. The school first established by the order at Nazareth, to provide religious education to the early Catholic settlers, became Nazareth Academy, a sort of finishing school for the young women who emerged from that frontier. If a German or Irish Catholic immigrant hoped to make his way up in the business world of Kentucky, Alabama, or Tennessee, he could send his young wife, and later his daughters, to Nazareth Academy to learn the social graces of a prosperous housewife. It was one of the first southern boarding schools for women, and gained the notice of strivers all over the region.

Inevitably, the convent adopted some of the style of a finishing school, enforcing a similar set of norms for the young novitiates. They did not ordinarily speak to professed sisters, unless they were in class or on special days. This rule was meant to give the young women discerning their vocation a chance to be private in their own thoughts, to communicate mainly with God. But in practice, it felt like an awful punishment, an enforced bottling up of everything they wanted to do and say and feel. They could not even say "Good morning," and were instructed to speak only at designated times or when absolutely necessary.

Just as Catholic high schools in the early twentieth century taught classes for girls in comportment and etiquette—how to stand up in a theater, how to behave on a date—the nuns in training were instructed that their vow of modesty included a certain grace and economy of movement. They were never to run up and down the steps.

They were always to move slowly, circumspect and propelled by prayerful intention.

They adopted this demeanor even with their families. The sister of one postulant remembered coming to see her on visiting day and waiting for her in the formal parlor of the convent at Nazareth. The postulant walked into the room in her skirt, cape, and nylon cap. (Only when she took her vows would she wear the starched cotton bonnet, and spend hours of her life ironing the delicate pleats.) Their younger brother came up for a hug—their family was so proud she had been accepted to this prestigious convent—but she told him firmly to sit in his chair. "Now, I can't hold you in my lap anymore," she told him solemnly. There was, in fact, no such rule, but she had taken it upon herself to make one up.

During the dark years of the Depression, the order was indispensable. Ann Sebastian sent her nuns to staff twenty-four schools in seven states, including four public schools in Kentucky that could no longer pay their teachers. She opened a camp for girls in Maryland and a mission to serve African Americans in Alabama, where no other hospital was willing to treat them. There were so many students and sisters coming and going from Nazareth that the order eventually had to widen the circular path at the entrance to the campus at the request of the Greyhound Bus corporation.

The Catholic Church in the United States, meanwhile, had turned its missionary gaze toward the east, to China and India. That was the new frontier; the Midwest had become a well-established center of Catholicism. The Sisters of Charity of Nazareth had an agreement with the Passionists since the early 1930s to begin a foreign mission in Asia, but the political turmoil in China, where many Catholic missionaries were already working, prevented them from accepting a post there.

In September 1931, Father Charles Cloud, the leader of the Jesuit Province of Chicago, made a trip down to Nazareth to ask them to consider joining the Jesuits in India. His priests had just been asked to take over a crucial mission in the North Indian province of Bihar, close to where Mahatma Gandhi was then organizing indigo workers against the British. Father Cloud came in person to make the request, but the mother superior and her councillor promised only to think about it.

By the time Ann Sebastian took over the leadership of the order in 1936, its original pioneering spirit had faded. The center of Catholic life in Kentucky had shifted from the historic settlement at Bardstown to Louisville, which became an archdiocese in 1937. Louisville had its own cathedral, with elaborate stained-glass windows built in the Arts and Crafts style, an embodiment of the city's wealth. Its patrons were the Brown family, owners of one of the most prominent distilleries in Bardstown.

The sisters made themselves useful to the elite of Louisville society. Ann Sebastian was not entirely comfortable in her highly scrutinized and powerful position. She used to say that Ann Sebastian was her "stage name." But she knew that the Sisters of Charity had a crucial role to play. They established a Catholic girls' school, Presentation Academy, where affluent families sent their daughters to be educated. (In the basement of the cathedral, they ran a night school attended by newsboys, bootblacks, and children laboring in the factories and shops.)

Ann Sebastian also turned her attention toward modernizing the Nazareth campus. The convent, built in 1854 in the antebellum style out of bricks fired on the grounds, was part of a sprawling compound, including the convent, a college and girls' school, dormitories, kitchens, and St. Vincent's chapel. But it had few comforts. The sisters still had to carry well water inside for bathing and cooking. In 1936, a new dam gave them a reservoir for water. The same year, the entire building was tuck-pointed, replacing all the old mortar to give the building the appearance of very fine joints between the old bricks. In 1938, construction began on a new infirmary building, and two years later, a renovation of the kitchen, including a new terrazzo floor. That same year, 1940, the Salt River Branch of the Rural Electrification Association finally agreed to extend reliable electricity to Nazareth.

After the December 7, 1941, attack on Pearl Harbor, Ann Sebastian knew the country would be drawn into the war, but she did not believe her order should be. Four days later, she gave her direction to the congregation: "Let us pray to the Immaculate Queen of Peace continuously until this awful conflict is over." She thought personal holiness, an example for other Christians, would be their greatest service. Six months later, in July 1942, when Ann Sebastian stood for reelection as superior, she made clear that her second term would be more of the same, an affirmation of her belief that meticulous attention to the order's daily rule was as important as their service to others.

She sent a letter to the congregation explaining her priorities: "To assure uniformity in wearing the habit," including minute details about the proper way to wear the cap, sleeves, and apron strings, which were all modeled on the dress of the pioneers. "To delete phrases not theologically sound" from community prayers. To "reaffirm restrictions" concerning the use of money, to limit their personal correspondence to four letters a month and limit their home visits to one day a year. (Those whose families lived far away could choose to have five days every five years.) And, most important, to "observe daily silence on the missions" just as they would while at the motherhouse. In other words, even when the sisters were sent out into the world, Ann Sebastian expected them to carry the prayerful silence and discipline of the convent with them.

This impossible standard was not so different from the ones imposed on other well-educated women in Kentucky at the time. The women who worked in the Curtiss-Wright aircraft plant or the Hub Tool Company of Lexington, as draftsmen in the naval ordnance plant, or as butchers at Fort Knox typically received uniforms suitable to the work—coveralls, shirts, and pants—but they dared not wear them outside the factory. They walked out of the factory doors wearing the same dresses they wore walking in.

Ann Sebastian became a bulwark against change; she wanted her sisters to continue their work and to be circumspect about the social changes rumbling through American society. She could see what was happening among women in the United States. The exigencies of the Depression and then the war had forced women into unfamiliar roles. They entered what was then called "public work"—a job outside the home—to sustain their farms through the Depression.

The memoirs of women of this period, the lay contemporaries of the young sisters serving the order at the time, reveal the thrill of tasting a life unlike anything they might find on the farm. The novelist Bobbie Ann Mason, who grew up on her family's farm in western Kentucky, remembers that her mother spent the war years running the enormous machines at a factory for men's suits, enveloped in the clouds of steam that billowed off the pressers. Her mother learned in that time "not to be afraid to be herself," Mason recalled. Violet Kochendoerfer, whose memoir of the war years was published by the University of Kentucky, hid her ambition behind a veil of patriotism. "I didn't join the Women's Army Auxiliary corps to help my country's war effort. I did it in selfish rebellion when my rise in the business world was thwarted because I was a woman."

The young Sallie Bingham, daughter of one of Louisville's richest families, the owners of *The Courier-Journal*, remembered the "extraordinary birds of passage" who occasionally blew into Kentucky in those years, like Nila Magidoff, the Russian wife of an American foreign correspondent. She came to the United States shortly after Pearl Harbor and barnstormed the country, alone, in a stylish mink jacket and hat, collecting old clothes to be sent to Russia. (Clementine Churchill had organized a similar charity drive through the British Red Cross.) It was the first time Sallie had seen a woman who was not poor but had no desire to conform to the stifling notions of what a lady should be. She became ever after that "an indication that there was another way."

When the war ended, the taste of independence sometimes turned bitter. Bobbie Ann Mason's mother welcomed her husband back from the war but found that he wanted nothing more than to return to his corn and tobacco and mules. She could not convince him to try factory work, and Mason's granddaddy and granny put a stop to her attempt to run a hamburger and catfish joint. "Ain't fitten work" for a married woman, they said. "I thought I saw a little go out of her then," Mason wrote. Sallie Bingham's mother spent the war years in her husband's chair at the newspaper, writing editorials twice a week that championed Roosevelt's foreign policy in Europe. His return ended her newspaper career. She went back to giving elaborate weekend parties, at which the list of entertainments—dinners, cocktails, and tennis—would be pinned to the guest-room curtains. "But something was lost," Sallie remembered. "And the newspaper became once again a kingdom of men."

This riptide swirled around the women of the Sisters of Charity as well, and there was little that Ann Sebastian could do to stop it. Their work in hospitals and schools was essential, and that impulse to serve the world by being fully part of it was strong among the younger nuns in particular. They were open with one another and with their families about wanting to fulfill the order's stated intention to take on an overseas mission.

The young nuns had some support within the order; it was not a monolith of conservatism. Nazareth College, a teachers' college, was led by Sister Margaret Gertrude Murphy, an ambitious nun with a PhD in theology. She wanted every woman who walked through the doors of Nazareth College to confidently take her place as a Christian woman in society, whether domestic, civil, or religious. Murphy pushed students and their parents to take the jobs available under the Works Progress Administration, and she wanted the college to be a scholarly institution, not a finishing school. She invited a classics scholar to give the commencement address in 1936 and, the same year, staged Euripides's *The Trojan Women*. In an effort to make the college more expansive and international, she wrote to church officials, embassies, and families in Mexico, the Caribbean, South America, and China, which was then an ally of the United States, asking them to send students to Nazareth Academy.

Ann Sebastian, on the other hand, did her best to keep the "worldly atmosphere" away from the community. She tried to turn the sisters' gaze toward the past. She turned Foundation Day, once a simple observance of the order's founding, into an elaborate celebration. She put her faith in the power of prayerful observance in everyday life, thinking that it would serve as a shield against change. What else but those rules defined who they were as a community?

The young women found ways to quietly subvert these rules. There was a phrase they could use when they wanted to speak out of turn or step out of the bounds defined for them: "Presumed permission?" It was meant as a question, to ask a superior whether they had permission to do so. The nuns in training used it all the time, whenever they wanted to talk to each other or complain, and they extended the idea as far as it would go, using "Presumed permission?" to run an errand and in the process give themselves an afternoon of freedom, with the cover that they had in fact followed the rules.

Ann Sebastian tried to rein in the use of "presumed permission"; she didn't like when it was interpreted too freely. "May I say that the matter of sisters going several places on a permission granted to take care of one errand is certainly lacking in regular observance," she wrote in one letter to the members of the order. When there were no other plans or tasks at hand, she felt that sisters should remain quietly in prayer rather than take the liberty of assuming they might go and do what they like.

On October 1, 1945, she wrote a circular letter saying she wanted to have "a little intimate talk" about certain points of rule: "promptness at prayers and meals; faithfulness to prescribed hour of recreation; use of radio and warning against unsuitable programs; attention to silence when prescribed, addressing others using refined social speech." It was those rules, she thought, that kept them together as a "regular, fervent Community."

Nevertheless, change would walk right into the heart of this community. In December 1945, two young Jesuits, Dan Rice and Jim Cox, arrived at St. Joseph's Infirmary in downtown Louisville, one of the flagship hospitals run by the Sisters of Charity. The end of World War II meant there was an opening in Asia, and a chance once again for the Chicago Jesuits to send missionaries to India. Before they could go, the young men had to be declared free of tuberculosis and healthy enough to withstand the cholera, malaria, and breakbone fever they would surely encounter. So they traveled the sixty miles from their seminary in West Baden, Indiana, an old luxury hotel that the Jesuits bought for a dollar during the Depression, to St. Joseph's. It was the closest good hospital, just over the Ohio River border in Kentucky. The young priests spent a few days with the sisters, chatting over Coca-Colas about their new mission to India.

Before the two Jesuits left, one of the sisters confided in Jim Cox, the quieter of the two, about her hopes. She wanted to go somewhere—China or India—and now that the war was over, she hoped it might be possible. He left her with a photograph of himself inscribed with a promise: "I'll be praying for the fulfillment of your vocation." And he carried her request with him on the long journey to India.

TWO

The Mission at Mokama Junction

T he East Indian Railway line stretched like a chain along the southern bank of the mighty Ganges River, linking Delhi and Calcutta, the centers of power of the British Empire. Between these two grand cities—Delhi, a playground to Mughals and viceroys, and Calcutta, a circus for traders and intellectuals—lay the vast riverlands of Bihar. The Ganges floods its banks each year, spilling rich silt into the farmland on the southern edge of the river. When opium and indigo ruled Bihar, traders floated their finished products downstream on barges from factories in Patna, the region's one big city, to waiting ships in Calcutta.

There is a turn in the Ganges about sixty miles downstream from Patna, a point where the river widens and slows. This became a natural resting point, or mokam, for vessels making the long journey. A bit of commerce sprouted here and grew into a small market town known as Mokama. There was nothing otherwise remarkable about it, but when the British laid their railroad tracks along the same route, following the Ganges from Patna to Calcutta, it was logical that they would put in a junction at Mokama, so trains running east to west could meet the line running south.

When American Jesuits first came to the area in the 1920s, it wasn't really a mission at all. The priests were railway chaplains who ministered to the employees of the East Indian Railway, and any other Catholics who happened to live near the stations at Mokama and two other nearby towns and wanted to hear Mass. Many of the railway employees were mixed-race Anglo-Indians. In the cruel subtleties of the colonial hierarchy, Protestant Anglo-Indians, who were often placed in the civil service, were slightly above the Catholics, who had their niche in the administration of the railways. It was unglamorous work in obscure places, but it was secure, and every railway colony—a little cluster of dormitories, a dispensary, perhaps a school and an officers' club—formed a tight-knit community, and the Jesuits did their best to serve them.

The Jesuits initially defined the Mokama Mission as a sprawling territory surrounding Mokama, more than five thousand square miles, stretching down from the Ganges as its northern border. The first priests who were posted there talked constantly about the potential to extend their mission beyond the existing Catholics to everyone else—"ad paganos." There were millions of people living here, the vast majority of them Hindus of every caste, with a large minority of Muslims and a sizable population of Indigenous groups in the forested areas of the interior. But the area was so vast, the populations so varied, and travel between the villages so difficult that they made little progress. Despite the urgings of their bishop to be more ambitious, they mostly settled for serving the Church in India as it was, shuttling between the railway colonies.

That began to change in the late 1930s. The people at the bottom of Bihar's hierarchy—the low castes like the chamars, or leatherworkers;

the "untouchables," or Dalits; and the Indigenous "tribal" communities, like the Santals—began to respond to the Jesuits' message. The priests in the mission weren't entirely sure why; perhaps it was the Jesuits' willingness to care for widows and orphans, perhaps the schools or the medicines they handed out, or perhaps a growing political consciousness that rose in tandem with the freedom movement. But they were finally making some progress.

When Marion Batson arrived in Mokama in January 1938, he was ready to devote himself to the difficult work of converting non-Christians and expanding the flock. At the time, there were about six hundred Catholics in Mokama and the surrounding area. For nearly a year he was alone, a wavy-haired American from Lincoln, Nebraska, living in a rented house near the Mokama post office. That house served as church, rectory, and mission headquarters all at once.

Before the Jesuits took over this property in the 1920s, it had been an old rifle range used by the British Army, not a particularly desirable property because it was so close to the commotion of the railway. The house suited Batson just fine, though, as it was just a few minutes' walk to the station—close enough that when the trains were late, as they usually were, he didn't need to wait for hours on the platform. He could just listen and bolt for the station as soon as he felt the ground rumbling and heard the chug and scrape of the wheels on the track. It was a straight shot north from the house, up the dirt path, past the railways workers' quarters and the locomotive shed, and then a shortcut across the tracks to the front of the station.

Batson worked mainly through catechists, local Catholics whom he trained and sometimes took on as employees and who would in turn educate other Indians in the faith. It was a complicated but necessary arrangement. India, then in the flower of its nationalist movement, had had enough of European missionaries. Indian leaders tolerated their presence as long as they served the public and were not seen to be directly proselytizing to non-Christians.

The earlier Jesuits had been content with their Christlike poverty; the missionaries rented rooms in the mud huts of whichever Catholic family might have them. Batson, on the other hand, had much bigger plans. Although he was the only priest in the mission for nearly two years, he opened mission stations every twenty miles, renting proper houses where the priests could live and work, and then building or buying permanent structures for schools along the railway lines and in the villages connected by them. He supervised the priests and paid the teachers and catechists. Some of them were earlier converts— Muslims or chamars who proselytized in their own communities. Others came from an older Catholic community in Bettiah, about 150 miles away, where generations earlier, a king listened sympathetically to a Belgian missionary, and he and his subjects converted en masse. Batson traveled constantly between the mission stations at Nawdah, Bihar Sharif, and Barh and sent monthly reports about his progress to the bishop in Patna. It was an expensive style of missionary work, but how else, Batson thought, could he show the people of Mokama that he was serious?

In June 1939, after less than two years of running the mission, he returned to the house after one of these trips to find a letter from the bishop waiting for him. He spent three days reading it over and over and then sat down at his typewriter to reply, furious that his superiors had dared to question the wisdom of spending thousands of rupees to win over the souls of Mokama.

"I have read it a number of times, and I must admit that I don't know what to do," he wrote. "From the day this sector was assigned to me, I have tried my level best to reduce expenses and still keep the work going on in each division. I have not opened up any new territory; from the first my plan has been to increase the number of Catholics in those villages where conversions had been made by my predecessors. I have tried to equip each of the four main stations with essentials needed for missionary life and work. I have tried to beg enough to support the whole work, but results have failed far short of the needed amount."

The Jesuits expected their missionaries to self-finance their work. Aside from a small stipend from the bishop, each mission had to ask for alms from the community that they served. The policy was meant to keep the priests faithful to their vow of poverty, to prevent any suspicion that they might be buying converts, and to make sure that new Catholics considered the Church to be their own.

Batson rejected that notion. He thanked the bishop for his generosity in covering his ever-expanding monthly deficits but balked at the demand to rein in expenses. "I don't see how the work can be curtailed nor the staff reduced without SERIOUS damage to the people recently converted," he wrote. "To stop work now will indicate to them that we were not serious in the beginning, that we have misled them, that they have made sacrifices at our suggestion only to be abandoned." He was livid at the request for "proposals" as to how he might economize. "May I suggest that some other missionary—able to support the whole work going on—be put in my place." He told them that he was deeply sorry, but "I can do no better than I have been doing." He implored his superiors to send someone else to take over this "impossible burden."

His threat to leave seemed to get their attention. His superiors came up with a new arrangement: they agreed to pay for the schools and the catechists, but he would have to fund the rest of his expenses,

and any extraordinary expenses such as land, by raising donations
from people in the area. "Retrenchment is a very hard thing," Bishop
Sullivan wrote, gently prodding him to control the mission's expenses.

Batson accepted those restrictions, but without a church and
proper mission house, he found it difficult to organize his work, to
keep track of the various converts and catechists, and, most important, to impress upon people that the mission had come to stay and
that those who joined the fold would be protected from persecution.
Batson seemed incapable of "retrenchment"; to pull back would be an
admission of defeat. And he was adamant about the need for land. "It
is impossible to have a school until they secure the rifle range, where
they can work undisturbed."

The bishop agreed to pay for land on which to build a permanent
mission: Batson arranged in April 1940 to buy five acres of land, the old
rifle range, from Her Majesty's Government for about seven hundred
rupees. In Bihar, land was everything. It signified permanence, a livelihood, and a clearly understood place in the region's intricate social
order. With that small piece of land and the mission buildings erected
upon it, Batson could signal to the people of Mokama that becoming
part of this Catholic community meant having a place to take shelter,
to bring your children to be educated and your dead to be buried. Permission to buy the land was contingent on the condition that it be used
for "educational purposes," so he began to build a boarding school for
boys, a way to educate the young in the faith and give their parents a
reason to trust the Church and want to be part of it.

For the next two years, this pattern repeated itself in the letters
sent back and forth between Batson and his superiors in Patna. Batson would spend his entire allowance, and then ask for more, in the
belief that adding more people to the payroll of the mission would
eventually pay off in conversions. His superiors would resist, he

would threaten to leave, and they would relent. Periodically, they visited Mokama to talk him down from his attempts to abandon the mission. At one point, he warned that if they refused to keep supporting his work, he planned to give his staff a month's notice to find other work and then "pile things up neatly for the big bonfire."

Batson refused to change. He was convinced, even after the beginning of World War II, that this was the best possible time for missionary work. The harshness of village life in Bihar, the daily toil to maintain a sense of dignity and hope, was made worse by wartime rationing and the conscription of thousands of Indian men into the colonial army. The Catholic Church, he believed, offered an alternative, an anchor of security and stability.

As the war escalated, it was no longer clear who was in charge in Bihar. The British administration had turned India into a source of raw materials, and colonial authorities were consumed by the fighting and supply shortages in Europe and North Africa. The independence movement had begun to splinter. Nehru and Gandhi had agreed not to resist the war effort, but other leaders saw an opportunity to assert their power while the empire was distracted. "The whole of India seems to be confused," Batson wrote. "Nobody seems to have a solution even to ordinary problems. Nobody seems sure of themselves."

Except for Batson. The Catholic Church, he insisted, should seize this moment. He believed that people were finally starting to trust the missionaries, because they were still there. They had weathered years of opposition from local political parties, who saw the Jesuits as little more than an extension of white rule by the British. The Jesuits had outlasted the Arya Samaj, Congress, the Hindu Mahasabha, the Kisans, and every other political movement in Bihar and managed to maintain support among the local population. "They think we must have the secret," he wrote. "To slow down now is to give up our big chance. . . . Now is the time to select our places and to gain a foothold." He imagined an independent India in which missionary men were leaders, building something out of the chaos. The bishop advised him to go out and raise funds and then do whatever he could manage. This, too, Batson rejected. The most important work was out in the field, he told them. Let others spend their days cultivating rich American and British Catholic donors.

His ideas grew ever more outlandish. He had plans for a much larger land purchase, for about four thousand rupees, to make Mokama "one of the best stations in the whole territory," once he had completed not only the school but also a medical clinic. One of his assistants had started a small dispensary, and he believed it had won over those who had earlier been hostile to their work. A few local merchants and landowners had donated some equipment for the school, but they wanted to make sure their money would not be wasted. They wanted to see the buildings finished before they would give more. Of course, Batson had nothing to show them; he didn't have funds to start construction. He hadn't even paid for the land. He had been cultivating a donor, but rather than ask him for the money to complete the purchase, he suggested that the Jesuits in Patna might raise some money from the United States to pay for the additional expenses and a few other debts he had piled up along the way. If he had something to show the donor, Batson figured, he might donate even more.

Faced with this latest of Batson's schemes—that the diocese should, in effect, engage in land speculation to indulge the whims of one rogue missionary—the Jesuits finally lost their patience. In a letter to Batson in November 1941, his superior, Father Loesch, admonished him, writing that he had lost "many hours of legitimate sleep" dealing with Batson's endless complaints and demands. Again and again, he wrote,

Batson glorified his high ideals but refused to see the danger in chasing them so recklessly. "You are apt to be discouraged by desiring to realize these ideals too fast."

Batson's troubles were of his own making, Loesch wrote. "You have repeatedly involved yourself in financial tangles by spending more on buildings and catechists etc than what you could reasonably expect." He spent more than other missions and yet had fewer converts to show for it. Worst of all, he had borrowed money from a member of his mission—the very people for whom he should have been an example of Christian rectitude—against the advice of his superiors. "Considering the manner in which you went into this transaction it is something definitely against the spirit of obedience and poverty as well."

They were angry, too, about the land he had purchased in Mokama. The final price was eight thousand rupees, twice what they originally agreed to spend. They were angry about the money they had been sending as a monthly subsidy for schools in the mission—schools that they realized had not yet been built—and they were angry that he dared to directly criticize his superiors in his letters. "Nor is it according to form in the Society to reprehend a superior regular and then send a copy containing such reprehensions to the Bishop." Loesch implored Batson to accept the guidance of those above him, even while conceding that obedience seemed to be against his nature. "I have noted that your spirit of independence revolts against such advice." He also beseeched Batson to consider the difficulty of running a mission when the war had made the Jesuits' presence in India even more tenuous. "Would that you understood the perplexity of financing the whole mission and the cares that arise out of the horrible world situation where hopes are slight that we will be able to continue the work as it has begun."

And yet, remarkably, Loesch did not cut Batson off. Instead, he accepted the obligation for the payment on the property in Mokama, although with the condition that the diocese would have to withhold "half of your alms in abeyance from next month."

There was one indisputable truth in all these criticisms: Batson was so absorbed in his own mission, fueling his work with drama and salesmanship rather than money, that he had little sense of the larger storm gathering around India. By the end of 1941, Batson was still trading angry missives with his superiors: at one point, he numbered the paragraphs of a letter from them so he could refute them, point by point. When the war reached the borders of India, he was caught unprepared.

Japan had entered the fight, and Britain was unable to defend its colonies in Asia. In February 1942, Singapore fell to the Japanese; in March, Burma followed; and in April, Japanese dive bombers hit Ceylon, the heart of Britain's naval operations in Asia. India was certain that it would be next. One newspaper in Bihar warned, "And as for defence, India is definitely much less prepared for it than Australia perhaps is. Her long coast-line along the Bay of Bengal will be at the mercy of the Japanese sub-marines, of Japanese naval craft, while Calcutta, Jamshedpur and other vital centres in North India will be within the reach of Japanese air-craft." Calcutta and the other ports on the eastern coast were part of the British supply lines, sending wheat and coal to troops in North Africa. Jamshedpur, one hundred miles west of Mokama, was Britain's biggest producer of steel.

Leaders of the independence movement were furious that the colonial government of India had agreed to plunge India into the war without even consulting them, but at Gandhi's urging, they pulled back their public demonstrations to show that they were not sabotaging a war waged in the name of freedom. On the surface, India appeared calm. But many Indians feared that they had been trapped into fighting for the losing side—for the very people who had kept them under colonial rule. They began to see the Allied effort not as a noble fight against fascism but, instead, as "an imperialist war with little in it for India" other than intense and worsening economic pressure. If India had been free, they thought, it would not be under attack.

It was not just fear that gripped Bihar, but anger and betrayal. Thousands of families in Bihar had sent their sons and fathers to fight in Burma—soldiers who were now caught in enemy territory with no clear way to get back home. Merchants in the big cities made plans to leave for the safety of their villages. Prices were rising, and anyone who had enough cash worth protecting poured it into the purchase of land, the only way to protect their assets from devaluation. Withdrawals from savings banks during the first three weeks of February 1942 were nearly double those in similar periods in preceding years. *The Searchlight*, the leading pro-independence newspaper in Bihar, argued that if the British were not capable of defending Malaya, they would surely do little more to protect India, especially not when there were threats in Europe and North Africa that were closer to Britain. "India has suffered and has been exposed to risk because its defence was related to and balanced against Imperial responsibilities elsewhere."

In Mokama and other cities in Bihar, this tension found its release in street violence. Amid the desperate grasping for political power, Hindus began to see their Muslim neighbors as targets. In the cities of Bihar, Muslims were often merchants who held wealth and property. In villages, they were usually laborers who occupied suddenly scarce and valuable land. Symbols of British rule, like the railway stations, were also targets.

The British, responding to the violence with further oppression, demanded an extra tax from every resident of the areas affected, supposedly to pay for the costs of providing additional security. It was merely punitive, of course, and many refused to pay it, so British authorities sent police into homes to confiscate whatever they could find—even brass cooking vessels—in payment. Europeans and Anglo-Indians were exempted from the tax, as were Muslims in certain areas and anyone who could show that they had actively assisted in the British efforts to restore order.

Batson tried to turn this to the advantage of the mission. He made applications and petitions, and wrote multiple letters of appeal to escalating levels of authority arguing that Christians in Bihar, like Muslims, should be exempt from the tax. They had been neither victims nor perpetrators of the violence, he wrote, and had complied in every way with the law. He invented a "Catholic Mission Authority" to give his letters more bureaucratic weight and wrote to the bishop asking for his prayers. "It will mean much to our work if we succeed." If he could defend "the Christian community" of Mokama against the unfair tax, Batson believed he could finally demonstrate the worldly advantages of belonging to the Church.

The British denied his request, but in the end, the war threw a savior into his path. On one of Batson's frequent train journeys between Mokama and Calcutta, he happened to sit next to Thomas Leslie Martin, the senior partner and chairman of the board of Bengal Iron & Steel. In 1939, the company had completed the construction of a new, modern steel plant in Calcutta, capable of producing more than 350,000 tons a year. It harvested the ore from the interior of Bihar and then smelted and refined it into the steel that would prove crucial to the British Army in Asia. By 1941, Martin's wife and children had fled to England for safety, and he was alone in India except for the company of his two Great Danes. A devout Catholic, Martin had made his fortune in India as a managing agent for one of the many commercial houses in Calcutta, descendants of the old East India Company. As the independence movement gained ground, the remaining British agents knew that their era was reaching its end. They had begun to take on Indian partners who would run these companies after independence, which seemed likely to come as soon as the war was over.

Martin wanted to leave something behind, a legacy other than having nourished the bones of the imperial war machine. Batson was happy to oblige him. He encouraged and indulged Martin's desire to construct an elaborate shrine to the Virgin Mary, with domes like the Hindu temples at Belur in the south, as a symbol of gratitude for her intercession. Martin was worried about the threat posed by the Japanese on the eastern front, Batson wrote. "It would mean MUCH to him if no invasion took place in India."

Of course, to build a shrine of appropriate grandeur, attractively set off against a lush field of green, Batson reasoned that he would need much more than just five acres. And with such a beautiful shrine, sure to attract many more souls, the mission would need the funds to complete the buildings for the boarding school and the dispensary. In June 1942, Batson wrote proudly to the bishop that Martin had agreed to pay for everything they needed—the land, the buildings, and the shrine.

But Batson was not satisfied. Martin's gift was the leverage he needed to finally be taken seriously by the local Hindu landowners, the people who really ran things in Mokama. In July 1942, he reported to the bishop that he had invited "our two wealthy zamindar neighbors," Ram Ratan Singh and Lilo Singh, to the mission house one evening for a chat. Batson delighted in his own cleverness: he told the two landowners that of course they would want to make a gift comparable to Martin's, in land or money, to show this British big shot that the wealthy of Mokama were just as magnanimous. "I also added that plans call for a nice big hospital east of the Rifle Range, near the shrine, and that a zenana ward or two must be donated by Lilo and another by Ram Ratan and another by Varma. They went away all smiles."

A maternity ward—a zenana is the women's quarters of a traditional family house—was "a magic word" in Mokama, Batson wrote. The powerful men of Mokama prized their male heirs, carriers of their privileged bloodlines, but they were powerless to protect their children or their wives against the fevers and complications that regularly claimed their lives in childbirth. In this way alone, they were no better than the lowest sweeper. Batson knew this, and so he promised them a "zenana hospital." Even if in the end it was nothing more than a small room with a bright red purdah, a cloth to separate it from the rest of the hospital, and the staff had no more skill than ordinary village midwives, "it will be something for them to get het [excited] about."

Lilo was the toughest to convince. Batson was sure that he could be impressed with "a bit of swank perhaps," and that the rest would follow suit. He described to the bishop his strategy: he had to be tough and assert his own authority. "They do not respect people who cringe or show any fear of them." This was the first time they had even entertained his requests. "I've beaten them on every score now, and they seem ready to play ball." Ram Ratan Singh paraded to the mission by elephant, suddenly resistant to the idea of donating land for the shrine. Batson threatened to go straight to the land acquisition office and buy it through the imperial authorities, the same way he had acquired the rifle range, and insisted that the only alternative was a gift.

By August 1942, Batson wrote to the bishop in triumph. "Feel like flyin' from here to Bar Bigha." He was ecstatic that his vision for Mokama would soon become a reality. Major construction would take time because prices were so high, but he was willing to wait for things to settle down. And Lahiri, the architect kept on retainer by Leslie Martin, had already managed to procure a supply of amber glass for the windows and then a shipment of nearly 2,500 bricks. Batson could at least make a start on building—never mind the monsoon, which soaked the roads as they began to give way under the weight of the carts bringing the bricks.

But it all unraveled in the fall of 1942, during the months of violence precipitated by the Quit India resolution in August. The Indian National Congress had asked for immediate freedom, an end to British rule in India. The British refused, and there began a wave of popular protests, which soon turned into violent attacks on any symbol of British rule. In Mokama, the police station was overrun, and the crowd attempted to kill the constables on duty. With the police overwhelmed, the looting moved to the trains and the warehouses at Mokama Junction without police interference.

Batson got caught in the fighting while he was away from Mokama in Kiul, a town on the eastern edge of the mission. He was attacked by a crowd—one of many incidents during the war in which white foreigners became objects of anti-imperialist anger. The railway tracks between Kiul and Mokama were destroyed, so he walked more than twenty miles back to Mokama Junction and arrived early in the morning of August 15, 1942, to find that the church had been ransacked. He had not seemed to realize how all his talk about a new shrine—on confiscated land, and built with the wealth of a British merchant—might appear to the people of Mokama. Hundreds of people swarmed the property, convinced there must be wealth hidden inside it somewhere. Of course there was nothing—just the gilt ciborium and tabernacle, which they stripped from the church. British and American troops came to "protect" the mission and made themselves at home, the old rifle range returning to its original purpose. The officers took over part of the priests' house at the mission, and Batson said Mass for them.

But Batson's grand plans were now indefinitely on hold. The colonial authorities, who were confronting both the threat of Japanese invasion and a serious local insurrection, were not about to hand over official title to land near a strategically important railway junction for the sake of an American missionary's eccentric dreams. The wealthy landowners would not give him money to fund a hospital on land he couldn't get title to. And he could no longer present himself to the people of Mokama as a beacon for the poor and oppressed; his mission had been taken over by soldiers, the same ones prosecuting this unwanted war.

For the rest of the war years, Batson did whatever he could to keep things moving. He met periodically with Lahiri, the architect. He tried to ingratiate himself with Martin, hoping to eventually get him to agree to fund the mission's work in other communities. But Martin was only interested in building churches, and Batson had no hope of acquiring more land. Batson crisscrossed Bihar by train looking for coal, which was in very short supply, and as food prices soared, his bills for rice ran into the thousands of rupees. He almost accepted an invitation to Karachi to conduct a spiritual retreat for the air force officers stationed there, so he could ask them for donations. But then he changed his mind. His place was in Mokama.

Batson saw what no one else could. He was convinced that the hospital, the one that hadn't yet been built, would be a breakthrough. Mokama had survived so much—the war, the nationalist movement, the riots. If he could just deliver this one thing, the hospital, he was sure that thousands of people would come into the fold. By April 1945, he was still waiting for possession of the land. The governor of Bihar even came for a visit, giving Batson the chance to talk up the planned hospital, but construction had been delayed for months. He could still hear the planes drone overhead, and he assumed that he would have to wait for the end of the war to get any relief.

By the end of the year, Batson seemed resigned. The war was over, but he was still waiting for approval of the land transfer. He went to Delhi and Calcutta to scrounge for army surplus supplies, and he began to lose faith in the future of the mission. "The present way is not sufficient. Our people are drifting away, becoming weaker instead of stronger in their faith." Without enough money, he could not maintain his catechists or pay enough teachers to keep the schools open. "Unless more vigor is shown," he wrote, it would be all but impossible to keep anything like a movement going among the chamars.

By early 1946, Batson was stuck. Without the title to the land, he could not complete the shrine or any of the other buildings. And without the school and the hospital, he believed he would never be able to make the mission self-sufficient. He went to the railway station to make one more trip to Patna to plead his case to Bishop Sullivan. The war was over, and there were some new American priests coming to Bihar. Maybe they would have some ideas.

THREE

A Plea for Help from India

One morning in March 1946, two priests came to see Mother
Ann Sebastian. Father O'Connor and Father McGuire were
both Jesuits sent from the provincial headquarters in Chicago. Ann Sebastian could not refuse to see them, but she dreaded the
meeting. O'Connor was a procurator of mission services, a fundraiser
and rustler of goods and people, a man whose job was to get whatever
the Jesuits needed for their missions all over the world.

Ann Sebastian knew what he had come for—sisters who could
help them. She entered the parlor with a cordial smile, but she was
determined, again, to refuse. Even with the war over, her nuns had
more work than they could handle. Every mail delivery brought letters requesting teachers for yet another new Catholic school in yet
another diocese, and not just in Kentucky. She had become adept at
writing warm, polite letters of refusal, but these two had come in
person, so she agreed to hear them out.

Her closest advisers in the order joined her, and they faced the two
priests as a united front. She asked them to sit down, but O'Connor

insisted on standing. He felt he could make his request more effectively that way. He came only as an emissary, he said, to deliver an
urgent request from Bishop Bernard Sullivan of Patna, asking the Sisters of Charity to join the Jesuits in serving the poor of Bihar. The
mission station at Mokama badly needed help, and the Jesuits were
looking for sisters with a "charism for risk"—an order whose founding principles moved them toward work in difficult places.

All they could do was ask; the Jesuits didn't have the power to
compel an order of religious women to work with them. Even the
bishop in Louisville—the highest authority in the archdiocese—
could only approve the decision once it was made. Orders of religious
women, even in the Catholic Church of the 1940s, maintained a certain degree of independence, and they guarded it jealously. They were
financially self-sufficient, and if they did accept a new mission, the
order would have to raise the funds to send their sisters overseas and
would be responsible for them once they arrived. So the Jesuits had
come to Nazareth as supplicants. The Sisters of Charity were known
as pioneers in Kentucky. Would they bring that same spirit to India?

Ann Sebastian gave him the standard answer: Of course, they
were ready to serve foreign missions. The order had agreed to do so
years earlier, and they already had an understanding with the Passionists to join them in China. However, with the new Communist
government there, the start of that mission seemed uncertain. Her
council members nodded in agreement. She was curious, though.
How had Bishop Sullivan, so far away in Patna, come to hear of the
Sisters of Charity of Nazareth?

O'Connor explained that Batson, on his last weary trip to Patna,
had met Dan Rice and Jim Cox soon after they arrived in India. Batson unleashed on them the most important sales pitch of his career:
he needed help in Mokama, sisters who could do everything—run

schools, hospitals, orphanages. Did they know anyone? Rice and Cox, fresh from their pleasant sojourn at the infirmary in Louisville, immediately thought of the nuns they met there. They were not only well qualified. As the young women had confided, they were eager to see the world outside Kentucky.

Ann Sebastian listened, but firmly said no. The angelus bell rang, and one of the sisters escorted the two visitors to see the chaplain. The mother general and her advisers joined the rest of the community. They began to talk again about Mokama, and gradually something pricked at Ann Sebastian's conscience. She looked at the young sisters murmuring around her—women whose ambitions she had so assiduously kept in check—and quietly admitted, "I think we've made a mistake."

Calling the priests back to the parlor, she tentatively agreed to send a few sisters, but not this year. They were simply stretched too thin. Perhaps they might send a few sisters next year?

O'Connor pulled out a letter from Batson inviting them to Mokama Junction and describing his years of planning and preparation. Even the building was ready for them. Moved, Ann Sebastian finally said, "Yes."

After all the years of conflict with his superior and the bishop, Batson had finally done something right. His last-ditch appeal had landed on sympathetic ears, and the Sisters of Charity agreed to come to India and carry out his improbable vision of the Mokama Mission. In the March/April 1946 issue of the *Patna Mission Letter*, the official newsletter sent by the Diocese of Patna to its member churches, its religious communities, and its supporters in India and abroad, Batson was given free rein to describe, in his best adventure-novelist style, his plans for Mokama. There was a photograph of a few newly arrived missionaries, including the two Jesuits from Indiana, Rice and Cox, whom Batson called "Rice and Curry." He reported his progress on the new buildings: a bungalow was under construction, and he was gathering materials to complete the hospital, although he graciously planned to wait until the sisters arrived before going any further.

He must have known that this particular newsletter would be read closely in Kentucky. He tried to entertain his audience with tales about the local fauna—the tasty varieties of pigeon that he called "squab," and the bullfrogs, scorpions, turtles, and lizards that were all put to use by the local healers as ingredients for "jungle" medicine. But Batson was careful not to alarm them too much. He mentioned that although the porters at the Mokama ferry landing were too scared to walk him to Mokama Junction at night, the night watchman was now feeling much better after adding two Alsatians to the bull terriers on duty with him. "Don't get the impression that Moka-meh is infested with thieves and brigands," he wrote. "The place is not exactly infested but they do grow well in these parts and thrive in spite of the night-watchmen." And there were two white owls roosting near the gate. He considered them a good omen.

For the rest of Bihar, March 1946 was dominated by the provincial elections, a reckoning after all the suppressed anger and suspicion during the war years. It was clear that Britain would not continue its imperial reign. But the colonial government was unable to come to any resolution of the fundamental question of who should represent an independent India. There were a host of political movements jockeying for power: the Indian National Congress, the self-styled statesmen of the independence movement, expected that they would simply take over the mantle of power from the British; the Muslim League wanted protection and assurances for the Muslim minority; various leftist parties, claiming to speak for urban and rural laborers, wanted political power that reflected their vast numbers; and a small but vocal Hindu chauvinist movement began to articulate its vision of a "pure" India, in which any "foreign" influence—British, Muslim, or Christian—would be expunged from public life. All these political parties were active in Bihar, and the elections would determine who controlled Mokama and the rest of the state after independence. Rather than try to bring these groups to agreement, the British officials who remained in India in 1946 (many had left for England soon after victory against Japan was declared) announced that they would hold elections in March to see whose vision of India the people actually wanted.

In Bihar, the dominant force was, of course, the bhumihars, the upper-caste Hindu landowners like Ram Ratan Singh and all the other men whom Batson had cajoled and flattered into making donations for the hospital. The bhumihars were the leaders of the Bihar Congress Party, but they had little in common with the leaders of the Indian National Congress, epitomized by the erudite, urbane Jawaharlal Nehru. For the bhumihars, land—*bhumi* is Sanskrit for land—and power were the only currency that mattered.

Nehru and the other Congress leaders in Delhi and Calcutta were the standard-bearers for Indian nationalism. They put on elaborate shows of support for the Indian National Army men who had been put on trial for "waging war against the king" for sabotaging the British war effort. But the men of the Bihar Congress had their own ideas about nationalism. The nation, in their view, was inherent in the land, and it belonged to those who were ready to spill blood to control it.

The bhumihars saw the March elections as a clear opportunity. They did not want to make any concessions to Muslims, even though they were a significant part of the population, and they had no use for the "secular" rhetoric of the national Congress leaders. By the end of March 1946, the bhumihar-dominated Bihar Congress Party won with an overwhelming majority. In many other parts of India, even though the elections restricted voting according to class status, a victory for Congress was seen as a victory for secularism, for keeping India together and united under the high ideals of Nehru and Gandhi. In Bihar, the Congress victory meant that the landlords' grip on power had tightened.

Winning the election hardened the lines between the bhumihars and everyone else. During the war and immediately afterward, there had been a huge transfer of land in Bihar: landlords ejected tenants and small farmers, buying their land and then renting it, sometimes to the same tenants, at higher rates. When land and food prices soared during the war, the landlords took full advantage, but none of this ever benefited the small farmers, who had to buy their food on the open market. Before, they might have claimed a tiny plot to till for their own use—a thin buffer against starvation—but now they had none. They had to work for wages, which the landowners could reduce at will.

There had been a time in Bihar when the subjugation of the lower castes came with certain obligations, a systematized version of noblesse oblige for bhumihars. According to the caste ideology of "jajmani" ties, the upper castes were bound, at least by tradition, to be the patrons of lower caste artisans and weavers, to show their piety and status by doling out favors, and to ensure that no one working their land was ever allowed to starve. Starving tenants signaled weakness to other landowners. But those traditional obligations had begun to fray.

Bhumihars began to push the tenants off the land, and the land grabs became worse as Partition approached. With the national government in utter confusion, only those who had clear title to the land could expect to keep it, and the bhumihars used the political power they had accumulated to claim as much as they could. This reconfiguration of land and people was an invisible but crucial change in the villages around Mokama. The same laborers were under the thumb of the same bhumihars, but now their position was much more precarious.

The land grabs were only the first ruptures to be set in motion as the empire began to fall to pieces. The next trauma was the threat of starvation. Bihar had barely recovered from a famine caused by the diversion of nearly all of India's wheat and rice to the war effort, when it faced a new food crisis after the war, a shortage of 8,500 tons per day. During the war, demand from the British war effort sustained India's industries—coal, cloth, and pig iron, and the Bata shoe factory, tannery, and wagon works in Mokama. As the war ended, the factories went idle, and the farm laborers who relied on those extra wages to feed their families had even less. The new Congress government called on paddy owners with a surplus of more than five hundred maunds (about twenty tons) to give up half of it to the ration authority, but almost no one complied.

One of the most vivid accounts of what happened in those early months of 1946, as the British Empire unraveled, is the memoir of Francis Tuker, a British Army officer who had been stationed in Bihar during the last years of the war. He witnessed the bitter consequences of all the forces pressing against the people of Bihar—the food crisis, the power grabs by the upper castes, and the instability caused by hundreds of thousands of decommissioned soldiers who were suddenly set adrift. After Partition, he returned to England and recorded his memories of the immediate postwar period.

Tuker noticed the early signs of a breakdown in civil order. Amid the food crisis, there was talk of famine. Factory workers in Bihar went on strike when their rations were cut, and by March 1946, the police joined them in a strike that spread across Bihar. The cause was economic: the cost and scale of rations for the police were not enough, given the high price of food and their paltry pay—only eighteen to twenty-three rupees per month (less than seven dollars). "It had always been a wonder to us that the police remained loyal," Tuker noted.

The strike also served a political purpose. It allowed the police forces to demonstrate their loyalty to the Congress leadership, who were likely to become their new masters, and it undermined the British civilian government. In May, in Patna, Saran, and Mongyr, Bihar's postal workers joined the police in striking, demanding more wages and allowances and obstructing the delivery of mail. The police would not respond to their colonial superiors' orders to keep the peace, and in some cases even demanded money to provide security. British officials considered sending out tanks, and they ordered troops to treat any crowd of people as hostile. Their authority was slipping away.

Meanwhile, nearly two million demobilized soldiers headed home. Indian soldiers had paid a heavy price in World War II: 24,000 killed, 64,000 wounded, 60,000 captured, and 11,000 missing on active service. They had fought and died in the Burma and Arakan campaigns; in Italy and Greece; and in North Africa and the Middle East. The average wage for soldiers was sixty to seventy rupees per month, and they would send most of it home—often just enough to keep their families alive. The British Army expected to shrink the Indian fighting force from 2.5 million men to 700,000 by the end of 1946, so they slowly began sending soldiers home to India from the Middle East, Burma, Malaya, Hong Kong, Japan, Borneo, and Siam.

Immediately after the war, there were high hopes among soldiers for a peace dividend. The British Army, in its recruitment propaganda, touted India's postwar prospects, promising soldiers that they would get jobs with India's new heavy industrial and transportation companies and that irrigation canals would make their farms more productive. None of this materialized, setting the stage for widespread disturbances among the armed forces. As soon as the war was over, the government decommissioned soldiers to remove them from the army's payrolls and reduce Britain's massive war debt.

Regimental headquarters turned into demobilization centers. The Rajputana Rifles Center, for example, demoted six thousand men and fifty officers, training them for animal husbandry, poultry farming, and basic accounting. But none of the newly decommissioned soldiers were able to find work. Unlike at the end of World War I, when soldiers were given land grants, those going home after World War II received fifty-six days' pay and 350 rupees as a parting gift, but no land, none of the benefits they had been promised, and no way to support their families as the price of food continued to climb. In some cases, soldiers returned home to find their families starving.

Tuker saw how this rapid and poorly executed demobilization sowed some of the seeds of violence. The decommissioned soldiers took the skills they had learned in the army and joined political militias or became bodyguards for politicians. It was not hard for them to find arms, for parts of Bihar and Calcutta had become unregulated ammunition dumps for the departing American army. "Now another problem began to appear: the surplus arms and ammunition of the United States Army," Tuker wrote. "We had had solemn promises that all of this would be completely destroyed so that it should not get into the hands of the lawless elements of India."

At one point, to verify whether those promises were being kept, Tuker sent some of his men to examine an American site just north of

Calcutta. Instead of an orderly disposal, they found about five thousand laborers exhuming sticks of dynamite and million of rounds of ammunition, "all unexploded and simply buried for anyone to find." The British Army, he wrote, managed to find and dispose of most of that cache. But some of it had already been claimed by scavengers who hoped to sell it for the brass and others who had plans for "more lethal purposes in Calcutta, Bihar and Punjab." As Tuker put it: "Many Indian men, women and children have since bitten the dust, holed by American ammunition."

The ties that bound landlords and tenants together were coming undone not just in Bihar but across India. In June 1946, the national Congress leadership proposed a law that would abolish "zamindari," the traditional feudal landowning system that had been supported and strengthened by British colonial law and administration. In theory, abolishing zamindari would end the exploitative relationship between landlords and tenants and allow tenant farmers to own the land they tilled. In fact, the landowners pushed the tenants off their land and in some cases forcibly stopped them from tilling that land, so they could claim it as their own under the new law. Many peasants reacted with anger and violence, and landlords organized in retaliation.

In Mokama, the bhumihars rose up on July 7, 1946. Fifty of them met and resolved to defend their hereditary privilege to the land. With the cooperation of the local police leaders, they issued notices to more than two dozen people under Section 144 of the Criminal Procedure Code, which prohibited more than two people from gathering on any disputed land, to prevent tenants from tilling the land. It required the land to lie fallow until the dispute was settled.

Peasants in villages all over Bihar, who faced retribution simply for trying to till the land that fed them, pillaged grain hoarded by landlords, formed themselves into guerrilla groups, breached landlords' irrigation bandhs, and cut wood from their forests. In some areas, Muslim and Hindu peasants joined hands against their landlords. The landlords, meanwhile, were so adamant in defending what they considered their rightful claims that in a few cases they brought women whom they otherwise kept in seclusion, in purdah, out into the open to help defend their land.

At this point, the British government and the army began talking about what they would do if they needed to make a hasty exit, reasoning that if the violence worsened, a step-by-step withdrawal might be worse. They planned to immediately grant independence to the areas that had not seen communal violence, to hand over the Indian Army to Congress rule, and to move British troops out through the Muslim-majority territory that would become Pakistan. Muslims, they thought, were much more loyal. They called it the "breakdown plan," to be used in the event of a total breakdown of order and open civil conflict.

India's "breakdown" began at the end of the summer of 1946, with Direct Action Day on August 16, a nationwide day of protest organized by the Muslim League to rally Muslims across India in support of their own, separate state. Despite everything that had already happened, many in the British armed forces believed that calm would somehow prevail, that this day of protest would pass as others had, without significant violence.

Tuker wrote that the British military at that point still viewed these rallies, strikes, and shop closings as tools used by political parties to mobilize their supporters around some new outrage. They thought of the violence that typically occurred during them as isolated and orchestrated, without deep roots in popular anger, and therefore unlikely to find purchase in the general population.

They miscalculated severely. Direct Action Day began with a show of strength by the Muslim League in Calcutta. It escalated into days of violence and retaliation in the city, in which hundreds of Hindus and even more Muslims died. The violence and calls for revenge spread to the countryside, and led to a notorious episode of violence against Hindu landowners in Noakhali on August 29. There was much more driving this: anger at Muslims, because of the Muslim League's unwavering support for the British during the war effort; the anger of Muslims, who felt betrayed by the British and fearful of the prospect of living under Hindu majority rule; and underneath all of this, the bitterness of people who had been pushed off their land, and the fury of those who had pushed them.

There are widely varying accounts of the atrocities of that period. Tuker described some of it: bodies that had to be cleared from sewers and water tanks; the "odd bodies in sacks and dustbins that were beginning to make themselves known" in Calcutta's Sobhabazaar market; a rickshaw stand found smashed to bits, with every rickshaw puller murdered and two children, wounded, found among them. There were at least 450 corpses cleared from the streets in Calcutta after those few days; the actual toll may have been in the thousands.

During the violence in Calcutta, Tuker's troops were in their garrison in southern Bihar, in Ranchi, with orders to "watch Bihar," in case any violence occurred there. Weeks passed, and nothing happened, so they waited. On the morning of October 16, 1946, "alarming reports suddenly appeared in the Hindu press" in Bihar—the newspapers controlled by the upper-caste landowners—of the violence against Hindus in Bengal, violence that was presumed to have been committed by Muslims. Tuker believed, although it was hard to say for sure, that those exaggerated reports set off the subsequent massacre in Bihar. The state had been quiet for weeks, but once the newspapers in Bihar took up this narrative of revenge, in which Hindus in Bihar were exhorted to avenge the violence against their Hindu brothers in Calcutta, the events of the subsequent days were all but preordained.

The violence moved through Bihar like a freight train. It began in Patna, with a series of stabbings of Muslims in the city. By October 31, forty Muslims were killed at Teragna Station. As the news of each episode moved along the railway lines, the violence gained momentum. It moved along the Ganges and then down into the interior of Bihar, following a path downstream like water during a flood. Sixty-three were found dead in Chapra. Then fifty in Bhagalpur, seven in Bihar Sharif, thirty in Khaira.

In a typical attack, a mob of several thousand people would surround a village, killing all the Muslims they could find. It wasn't hard to know who they were; their neighbors identified them, or they could be recognized by their clothing. In many villages, the Muslim population was reduced to "nil," according to the notations made by civil servants who were sent to record the extent of the violence once it was over. In the span of a few weeks, more than 7,000 people, almost all of them Muslims, were killed in Bihar in systematic purges, village by village. Kanchanpur village, for example, had a population of 1,079 Hindus and 309 Muslims in August 1946, according to the notes in Tuker's records. The area had not seen any communal violence in more than twenty years. A survey of the village weeks later found that there were no Muslims remaining in Kanchanpur—about half had been killed and the rest had fled.

The violence was not random. It was carried through Bihar on the shoulders of the powerful: first by Hindu traders in the towns, who avenged the attacks on their counterparts in Bengal by organizing violence against Muslims in Patna, and then by the zamindars, the landowners in the countryside. They called together their Hindu tenants, spreading the news of violence by Muslims, and in some cases provided the arms used in the attacks that followed.

Making things worse, there were not enough troops left in Bihar to stop the violence; most had been diverted to Calcutta. "Bihar had been skinned of its battalions," Tuker wrote. The railways were so crowded with troops moving east toward Calcutta that by the time Tuker got the order to move west with his regiment into the villages closer to Patna, he could only move his troops by road. "Ranchi to Patna by road was 280 miles; at Ranchi were the reinforcements, around Patna the trouble."

Tuker had very little ability to communicate with his superiors as he tried to move his troops across this territory, "fourteen thousand square miles of half-flooded land." Whoever was organizing the violence had also made sure to attack the railway tracks and to cut the telegraph and telephone lines. Civilian operators, too, became targets. The Indian women in the Women's Auxiliary Corps and British and Indian soldiers stepped in to keep some of the lines open, repeatedly repairing them after each round of sabotage.

With communication interrupted, Tuker and his officers had no way to know where they were most urgently needed. They moved their men for miles around tiny villages, chasing after slaughter, but almost always arriving too late to stop it. Forward patrols reached villages after the killings had already begun, and all they could do was help rescue the people fleeing. Troops arrived in villages to find all the houses burned, the bodies of Muslims with them.

Tuker received a report from one of his colonels describing the scale of the violence surging through Bihar: "He estimated that his men had brought in well over twelve thousand Muslims from an area of about one thousand square miles inhabited by half a million Hindus who were determined to exterminate the eighty thousand or so Muslims." In effect, within a week, there was a wholesale ethnic cleansing of these villages, with Muslims escorted out by the British Army.

By November 3, the situation had become so dire that Nehru and the viceroy felt compelled to visit Bihar to assess the damage and try to calm things down. In three months, from October to December 1946, more than four hundred thousand Muslims were either displaced or directly affected by violence. About fifty thousand of them left Bihar entirely for Bengal. Others were forced to leave their villages and make their way by train or by foot to the relative safety of Bihar's towns—Patna, Chapra, Mongyr, Bhagalpur, Gaya.

This marked the beginning of the movement of Muslims out of India's interior; although Partition itself had not yet happened, these were also people displaced by the same political forces that would later remake the subcontinent. These were the internally displaced, people whose villages had cast them out, so they had nowhere else to go. Muslim League volunteers escorted many of them out of Bihar to Punjab and other areas.

This massive movement of people caused disturbances that rippled throughout India. The trains were overwhelmed, and amid the constantly circulating rumors of ruptured train lines, factory workers, government clerks, and teachers could not get to work and their offices and factories had to close. Groups of refugees began turning up at railroad stations, clustering together for their own safety. But with so few trains available—they were still being used to take troops out to Bengal—the refugees began to camp wherever they stood, without any provisions for clean water or sanitation.

Mokama Junction was one of these crossroads, and inevitably, cholera took hold. The Jesuits were still there, along with a few staff from the railway hospital. They set up a makeshift camp near the railroad station—away from the platform, close to the banks of the Ganges. They didn't have hospital beds or equipment, so they lined up charpoys, or string beds, in the open air by the river. They had no nurses—the sisters from Kentucky would not arrive for months—and there were not nearly enough doctors. Anyone who was well enough to leave had already done so. A desperate message reached the superintendent of the medical college in Patna, so he sent a few doctors and a handful of medical students to Mokama.

Dr. Dilip Sen was among the student volunteers. His father was a civil surgeon in Bihar, and Sen had carried on the family tradition, attending Patna Science College and then the prestigious Patna Medical College. Everyone in the city of course knew about the protests, but the violence interrupted his studies that fall only for about a month, when things were in such turmoil that the students were told to stay home. About once a fortnight, British troops marched through the town to keep the peace. He heard from his father that there were injured soldiers being treated at the hospital by the civil surgeons, but they were kept under close guard, so he never saw them.

Sen had read about riots in the newspapers—there were brief reports about incidents all over Bihar—but it was only when he arrived in Mokama that he realized the extent of the violence. The purges had convulsed the villages and sent waves of people onto the trains. When the trains stopped running, there were a few buses, but unless people were healthy enough to travel by foot, it was almost impossible to move in and out of Mokama. The sick poor were left behind.

Nearly all of them had diarrhea; those who tested positive for cholera were sent to the open-air camp. Sen and the other medical students and doctors tried to rehydrate them with saline drips given intravenously, but for most of the patients, there was little they could do to help. The illness liquified their insides too quickly. Hundreds of people were left languishing on the charpoys; most of them died.

Dilip Sen lived just sixty miles away from Mokama, but if he had not witnessed the suffering there firsthand, he might never have known about it. It took days for word of a slaughter in a village in Bihar's interior to reach the newspapers in Patna, if it surfaced at all. It's possible that for him, as for so many others in India, the trauma of the months before Partition might have remained in the shadows of memory.

So perhaps it is not surprising that there is very little indication in the archives of the Sisters of Charity of Nazareth that the sisters in Kentucky knew what was happening in Bihar. In May 1946, as the food crisis, the land grabs, and the political turmoil were gathering strength, Ann Sebastian formalized the agreement to send members of her order to work with the Patna Mission. She hoped to inspire the young women with word that their long-deferred desire to serve overseas would finally be fulfilled. She sent a letter to the entire community, using language that reveals how far removed the convent in Nazareth had become from the devastation in Asia. "And now for the atomic bomb! We are entering foreign missions. The Patna District of India!"

Batson's quixotic project at Mokama was about to become a reality, and the sisters relied on him and the other Jesuits for news. There is no indication that they knew the extent of the violence or what had caused it. They did not realize the problems Batson might have created for them by soliciting cooperation and donations from the powerful bhumihars, for an institution with the stated purpose of serving the poor and the dispossessed. They didn't realize how little support they would have once they reached Mokama, with the population and the local administration spent and traumatized by violence.

They did, however, hear about the cholera outbreak, a clear call back to the order's history. In 1832, a cholera pandemic that had begun in Asia and had already moved through Europe reached the United States and eventually hit Louisville, where the order had just opened a small school and convent. Catherine Spalding, the founder of the order, crisscrossed the city to the homes of children who had been orphaned by cholera, gathering them up and walking with them to what would become an orphanage in downtown Louisville. Many generations later, her actions would be immortalized in bronze in downtown Louisville, in a statue of a striding nun in a Kentucky sunbonnet, carrying a child in one arm and holding another one by the hand.

This was something they knew. Another river, another abandoned people, another moment in which the women of Nazareth could prove themselves as true pioneers. Those who were chosen for the mission to India would have to be willing to say goodbye to their families and their lives in the United States forever. That message traveled by mail and flew by word of mouth to the sisters running schools, colleges, hospitals, medical clinics, orphanages, and convents. Ninety of them volunteered.

FOUR

The Moment of Freedom

Ann Roberta Powers was only twenty-one and teaching first grade at Holy Name School in Louisville when she heard that her order had finally accepted a mission overseas. The school year was over, so she was in Nazareth, at the motherhouse, to help with the annual "ladies' retreat" for Louisville's Catholic society matrons.

All the young sisters were talking about the new mission. Did you volunteer? Are you going to? Ann Roberta wasn't sure exactly how things were done, but she knew she wanted to go. As she prepared to leave the convent to go back to Louisville, having put on her black traveling bonnet over the white one, she met Mother Ann Sebastian coming down the stairs. "If going to India depends on volunteering, put my name down in your little black book," Ann Roberta told her.

Later, she sent a letter home to her parents to let them know that the order had asked for sisters to go to India and that she had volunteered. "But don't worry, they're not going to send me. I haven't made my final vows yet."

Ann Roberta had grown up in Cloverport, a town of about fifteen hundred people on the Ohio River. She was the eldest of ten, and the riverbank was like their front yard. The town had a few farms, a few stores, a post office, public schools, and a Catholic primary school, St. Rose's, which all the Powers children attended.

There wasn't really any industry in Cloverport, however, so most of the men had to leave town to find work. Some took the ferry to the General Electric plant across the river in Indiana, while others headed to the tar springs nearby, the source of a quick-burning type of coal that was exported outside Kentucky and had been used, legend has it, for Queen Victoria to heat her castles.

Ann Roberta's father was a carpenter, and her mother spent her days cooking and taking care of the house and children. Ann Roberta was born in 1924, so her parents raised their ten children during the Depression. They never did talk about it, but she knew her family was lucky compared to some others, like the neighbor boy who would usually end up at their breakfast table because his parents left him to fend for himself in the mornings. They had fish from the river, fruit trees, and a big vegetable garden. Even though they didn't have a freezer, they could keep their produce canned for the winter and would only have to buy the staples—flour, sugar, and coffee—with whatever her father earned doing odd jobs. Everything else they grew themselves.

When Ann Roberta was in the fourth grade at St. Rose's, a missionary who had been working in Fiji came to the school for a visit. He told them about his work on that remote island and the unusual mix of people who lived there—people from India and all over the South Pacific. Something about India fascinated Ann Roberta, and from then on, her family would tease her about this peculiar obsession with a country on the other side of the world. She wasn't sure how, but Ann Roberta felt sure she would get there eventually.

In April 1947, several months after she added her name to that little black book, Ann Roberta received word that she had been chosen to join the mission to India. She was the youngest of the group. There were two others who were also in their twenties: Ann Cornelius Curran, twenty-four, an operating-room nurse at St. Joseph's Infirmary, and Florence Joseph Sauer, twenty-eight, a nurse at Mt. Saint Agnes Hospital in Louisville. Two more were in their forties: Crescentia Wise, forty-seven, a nurse and pharmacist at St. Joseph's, and Charles Miriam Holt, forty-two, a teaching supervisor at a school run by the convent in New Hope. Their leader was Lawrencetta Veeneman, fifty-one, an experienced administrator at the convent who, reaching the end of her career, had returned to her first love, teaching music, at a school in Frankfort.

Ann Roberta's parents and siblings were not surprised by the news. She had been talking about going to India for so long. Her father did not stand in her way, but he found it difficult to accept the idea of his eldest child going so far away. "There are more than enough people in that nation to take care of themselves," he told her. "You're not needed."

But Ann Roberta felt sure that she was needed out there in the world, just as the men in her family had been. One of her brothers had served during the war, and he had been asked to stay in Japan for a year after the surrender. He would sit on the porch swing in the evenings, but never wanted to talk to his sisters about what he saw. "Girl, you don't know what it was like."

Their father, too, had served in his own way. During the war, Everett Powers was one of about fifty men from their town who would take a yellow school bus every day to Fort Knox, to help build a barracks for prisoners of war. The British were having trouble dealing with the large numbers of POWs taken by Allied forces. American ships would go to Europe and North Africa with supplies and return with POWs. There were two POW camps in Kentucky, and then another one opened at Fort Knox to deal with the overflow.

Everett hated that job. He had to be lowered feet first in a harness into a pit deep in the ground, where he worked alongside the prisoners. He became close to one of them—Spinelli, an Italian, who told him about the poverty and desperation of his family in Italy. Everett helped Spinelli buy shoes for his mother and sent them by mail, one at a time, so they wouldn't be stolen. Spinelli was an artist, and when the war was over and the prisoners were released, he gave Everett a painting he had made while he was imprisoned: a lighthouse at the top of a hill. Everett kept it, with pride, in their house on the river.

When it came time for Ann Roberta to prepare to leave, she did not hesitate. She had read Batson's wonderful letters describing Mokama—the building that would become the hospital, with rooms for the sisters on the second floor, the gardens and the verandas surrounding it. Everyone in the order had thrown themselves into fundraising—it was up to them to raise the money to pay for all the missionaries' expenses—and every sister was expected to do her part, especially the ones who had been chosen for this rare opportunity. Ann Roberta appealed to everyone she knew for support. Most of the people in the parish where she was teaching were Louisville railway workers, who proved to be extraordinarily generous. Cloth was still being rationed, but the women of Holy Name, the parish where she was teaching, found enough white cotton to sew all the habits the sisters would need for the first year. Two of them used old cotton flour sacks to sew Ann Roberta's underwear. The monsignor took a collection to pay for Ann Roberta's passage on the ship. She happened to answer the door of the parish office one day when a man, covered in soot and oil, came to hand over his contribution. "Here, sister, this is what I can give."

A few weeks later, on August 15, 1947, Ann Roberta and the other new missionaries walked down the wide steps in front of the mother-house in Nazareth. They had last used this grand entrance, with its towering neoclassical pillars, on the day they took their vows. After that, they were allowed to use only the side doors, a symbolic reminder that they had entered the community for life. They stopped and posed for a photograph against the wrought-iron railing—kindly Lawrencetta, Ann Roberta with her wide smile, gangly Florence Joseph in the back next to the delicate Ann Cornelius, stout Crescentia, and Charles Miriam, standing awkwardly with her eyes closed.

With each step, the order came closer to becoming a "mission-sending" community, one that went out into the world and faced the unknown. Ann Roberta accepted a gift, a small wooden "mission cross," and she listened to the priest, whose homily connected the work she would do to that of the French missionaries who had first ventured out into the Kentucky frontier. The entire congregation then recited the itinerarium, a prayer for the journey: "Be Thou unto us, O Lord, a help when we go forward, a comfort by the way, a shadow from the heat, a covering from the rain and the cold, a chariot in weariness, a refuge in trouble, a staff in slippery paths, a haven in shipwreck."

After the farewell ceremony, Ann Roberta went home with her mother to see her family in Cloverport. Her youngest sister, Gussie, was only four months old. It was the first time she saw her, and she assumed it would be the last. The war and the years that followed had marked everyone in the family, including Ann Roberta. Her sister

Marion said of her later, "The world was changing all of that time, and she was changing with it."

At the same moment, eight thousand miles away, India woke to its stained, blemished dawn. On the night of August 14, 1947, the British flag had been lowered, marking the end of colonial rule. In villages far removed from the upheaval, the night was pierced by bursts of firecrackers that children would remember decades later.

In New Delhi, statesmen tried to capture the weight of the moment in a few words. Jawaharlal Nehru implored his countrymen to embrace the future, to run toward the vast and dangerous unknown: "And so we have to labour and to work, and work hard, to give reality to our dreams. Those dreams are for India, but they are also for the world, for all the nations and people are too closely knit together today for any one of them to imagine that it can live apart."

In Bombay, the evening was jubilant and bright with anticipation. The alleys had been swept clean, there were bunting and streamers hanging everywhere, and floral arches spanned the wider avenues like rainbows. People went home early to bathe and change clothes, as if for a holy feast, and office workers laughed and chatted in the streets, ready to celebrate.

One young journalist attended a private celebration at the Taj Hotel hosted by the mayor. "At our table was a young Moslem Begum, a Hindu Congressman, a Parsi jeweler, a Polish Jew and his English wife, an American couple, Nehru's younger sister, a couple of newspapermen, one of whom was my host's son, and an industrial magnate—the half-French, half-Indian head of Tatas, J. R. D. Tata." He thought of his servants gathered at home. "They had pooled their rations, bought chickens to make a rice pilau and a large salmon, which was dressed with onion and garlic."

At midnight, the room was darkened and the new flag was illuminated. As the lights came on, everyone in the room—all of them now free Indians—greeted one another with fond embraces. The journalist took a moment to watch the scene outside from an open window. In the harbor, the ships tossed their searchlights across the water, and a solid mass of humanity came together in the open plaza between the Taj and the Gateway of India. He heard a few Englishmen singing "Auld Lang Syne" and "Jai Hind" to the tune of "Tipperary," and then he turned back to the crowd inside. "I noticed an elderly Hindu, wearing a red and gold turban, joining his hands in namaskar and bowing humbly to the flag. Then he sat down in his chair and wept." The next morning, it began to rain, and the downpour continued until late afternoon, drenching the parade of horses, soldiers, guns, tanks, men, women, and children.

FIVE

Aboard the *Steel Executive*

The mother general, in her wisdom, had split up the six sisters into two groups. It was cheaper than trying to find one cargo ship with room for all six of them. Left unsaid was the possibility that if something should happen to the sisters on one of the ships, at least the others could carry on with the mission. The first group of three sisters—Lawrencetta, Ann Cornelius, and Crescentia—boarded in Washington, then went to Philadelphia and Baltimore, where their ship, the *Steel Vendor*, was loaded with two thousand tons of sugar—a process that took three days—and then one more day in Philadelphia. The second group was booked on a ship leaving from New York. Mother Bertrand accompanied Sisters Ann Roberta and Florence Joseph on the train to New York from Kentucky. Charles Miriam came by herself from South Boston, where she was visiting her family.

Sister Charles Miriam Holt was forty-two years old and rarely went to Boston; she hadn't lived there since she was twenty-one. She entered the convent in 1927, and for twenty years she had gotten one day of leave every year. Most sisters saved up those days, waiting years until they could accumulate a week of time off—enough to make a trip home worthwhile. When Charles Miriam and the other new missionaries received word that they would be given three weeks to visit their families—a lifetime's worth of leave—they all understood why. They did not expect to see their families again.

Three weeks! What would she do with so much time? Her mother was old, her father long passed. When she got back to South Boston, things were much the same as when she left. Her brothers and sisters still lived within a few blocks of St. Eulalia's, where they had all gone to school. Their children—her nieces and nephews—ran in and out of one another's houses at lunchtime. They ate well; her brother Edmund was a butcher at Faneuil Hall.

The Sisters of Charity of Nazareth ran the school at St. Eulalia's, so when Charles Miriam had felt the call as a young woman, it was natural that she would join them. The order sent her to Kentucky, where she trained at Nazareth Normal School, spent five years teaching middle school in Henderson and Culvertown, then five years as a principal in New Hope. She was the only one of her siblings who left home.

Soon after Charles Miriam arrived in Boston, she got a call from St. Patrick's to fill in for a teacher who was ill. The weeks passed quickly. She spent most of it in the classroom but managed to make one last visit to the dentist. Leaning back in the chair, she revealed her big news: She was going to India! The dentist was delighted. He insisted that she get in touch with his brother, who worked for RKO Pictures in Bombay. It seemed unimaginably glamorous. RKO, run by none other than Joseph P. Kennedy, was the studio that had produced *Gunga Din*, *King Kong*, and *Citizen Kane*. She explained to the dentist that her ship would be sailing to Calcutta, not Bombay, but she carefully wrote down the name just in case: Charles O. Julian. She was from Boston, after all, and it never hurt to have a personal connection to the Kennedy empire.

A few weeks earlier, one of the other sisters in Kentucky had written to her aunt, a nun who belonged to a cloistered order, the Sisters Adorers of the Precious Blood, in Sunset Park, Brooklyn. She asked, could the cloister possibly accommodate three of the India-bound sisters for a day or two before they left? And so it was that Charles Miriam, Florence Joseph, and Ann Roberta spent their last night in America in a monastery in Brooklyn.

On the evening of October 27, 1947, the sky over New York Harbor turned a brilliant red, gold, and pink, filtering through the black wrought-iron gate of the cloister. Charles Miriam prepared to sleep in one of the guest rooms. She kept the piece of paper from Dr. Julian close, along with her rosary. At midnight, she heard the cloister rising up. This was how the Sisters Adorers earned their name—every night, they spent an hour venerating the Blessed Sacrament, a gesture to honor Christ's blood and sacrifice. She woke up to join the others. They had all been instructed to wear their black traveling habits, and Charles Miriam arranged the fabric carefully over her stout frame. A few hours later, they all stepped into a taxi and drove to the Brooklyn waterfront.

Between 1941 and 1945, American shipyards built more than five thousand vessels. In the last months of World War II, when it became clear that the Allies would emerge victorious, the U.S. War Shipping Administration began to plan ahead, commissioning ships, often combination cargo and passenger vessels, that could be converted to civilian use when the war was over. One of them, christened the *Sea Lynx*, was a 492-foot-long behemoth capable of carrying 17,000 tons of cargo, and the American government spent $3.5 million to build it. After the Allies declared victory in Europe in May 1945, most of the

American fleet was diverted to Operation Magic Carpet, which brought 3.5 million servicemen back to the United States by December of that year. But the *Sea Lynx* was delivered on November 21, 1945, too late for that task, so Isthmian Lines of New York bought it in 1946 and rechristened it the *Steel Executive*.

Mother Bertrand had been carefully checking the shipping news in *The New York Times* for days, and the *Steel Executive* was scheduled to depart on October 28. When the taxi arrived at the pier, Charles Miriam and the others walked up to the deck. A cluster of people had gathered to see them off: Mother Bertrand and her sister; a few priests; a few of the nuns from the cloister; and a contingent from the order in Boston, along with one of Charles Miriam's brothers. Someone had brought along a camera, and the young sisters— Ann Roberta and Florence Joseph—couldn't help but mug for the pictures, fooling around with the captain's wheel on the deck while they said their farewells.

Charles Miriam went belowdecks to explore and was pleased with the roomy shared cabin. It fit their three trunks easily, plus a dressing table big enough to make do as an altar for daily Mass. One of the ship's waiters came by to show her the kitchen where she could get coffee and sandwiches, and another steward adjusted the transistor radio. The two younger nuns compared their cabin to their berths on the Cincinnatian, the new B&O passenger train that had carried them across the Midwest to Baltimore. Olive Dennis, the first female member of the American Railway Engineering Association, had designed the interiors, which had comforts unlike that of any other train in the country—reclining seats, individual window vents, and ladies' dressing rooms stocked with paper towels and liquid soap. The two young women had never before ventured far from Kentucky, and Charles Miriam was amused at how dazzled they were by every step of the journey. Before the three sisters retired for the night, Charles Miriam had a word with Father Wyss, one of two priests traveling on the ship, about the schedule for Mass the next day.

Early the next morning, Charles Miriam woke to the sound of Florence Joseph's booming, exasperated voice. We're in the same place! she yelled. Charles Miriam looked out of the porthole and realized that the ship was still in New York Harbor—they hadn't moved at all. She had slept soundly, assuming they were on their way. But it took another day for the ship to be sufficiently loaded with cargo to make the trip worthwhile. When it was finally being nosed out of the harbor by tugboats, Charles Miriam kept a weather eye out for the Statue of Liberty. Soon, it loomed into view. It was cloudy, so she couldn't see it very well. The skyline, too, was obscured, but she could make out the line of the statue's outstretched arm and the curves of her torch.

Charles Miriam thought to herself, Who knows if I'll ever see these shores again? She said a prayer, for her own country and the one that would soon become her home. Still, she couldn't escape a feeling of unease. Why had she been chosen for this great honor and challenge? There were plans to open a school on the site of the hospital, but until then, she didn't know what she would be doing in India.

Before boarding the ship, Charles Miriam had little in common with the two young women she would be traveling with. Florence Joseph was only twenty-eight; Ann Roberta was even younger, twenty-two, and hadn't taken her final vows. Charles Miriam and Ann Roberta had gotten to know each other a little bit during the three weeks they spent together at St. Joseph's infirmary in Louisville in September. They learned how to take blood and urine samples and understand the basic tests. Florence Joseph was working as a nurse at St. Agnes nearby. And they had all been together for the grand departure ceremony, the parties and prize bingo matches during their last few days at the motherhouse in Nazareth.

Eventually, the ship picked up speed—to seventeen knots an hour—and moved out of the harbor. The sisters listened to Ann Roberta's transistor radio; they could still get the Sacred Heart broadcast, the same one they listened to in the evenings in the convent, even two hundred miles out to sea.

As the *Steel Executive* traveled the tedious length of the Atlantic, heavy rain made it impossible to walk the decks, and storms threw water against the porthole with furious impact. For days, the three nuns stayed in the cabin trying to keep the seasickness at bay. At one point, miserable with nausea, Florence Joseph vowed to get off the boat at the first port of call and stay there. The steward brought her grapefruit and crisp crackers, and Charles Miriam was touched by his thoughtfulness in the face of Florence Joseph's outburst; all of the stewards on this ship were so kind. When she sat down for dinner on the first night and laid her napkin on her lap, Charles Miriam noticed the napkin ring, inscribed with her initials.

A week into the journey, the sun broke through. The sisters started to spend more time above deck and got to know the other passengers, who were all returning to the subcontinent after waiting out those terrible months around Partition. There had been so much uncertainty about what would happen after independence, and whether the British and Americans who had been living in India would be allowed to stay. But the fears about a surge of attacks on foreigners proved to be largely unfounded—theirs were only a few drops in the ocean of bloodletting—and the passengers on the ship were among those who had chosen to go back: Father Wyss and the other priest,

Father Holland, to their missions in Calcutta; an American family, the Burtons, were traveling with two toddlers to Bombay, where Mr. Burton worked for an American oil company that hoped to gain a foothold in the Indian market; and a young couple, the Fonsekas, who were headed home to Colombo, Sri Lanka. Obliging and resourceful, Mr. Fonseka was the nuns' favorite. He couldn't keep their names straight, so he called them Prima, Secunda, and Tertia, in order of age. And he was full of practical advice about traveling.

His warm reassurances were a balm to Charles Miriam, who spent most of her time worrying. She worried about her rosary, which had been lost somewhere between the monastery and the ship. She wished she had packed a dictionary to settle the silly arguments about spelling or arcane historical facts that inevitably seemed to come up as the three sisters passed the time talking and exchanging trivia. Why hadn't she thought to bring one on the ship? Would it turn out that their dozens of boxes were packed with other useless things? She worried about the laundry that remained damp even after days of hanging on a line in their cabin. And she worried about her weight. Charles Miriam weighed more than 180 pounds, and if she ate everything on the menu, she thought, she wouldn't be able to get down the gangplank when they finally reached Calcutta. When Captain Green invited the passengers on a special tour of the engine room, with its massive boilers and turbines, Charles Miriam felt awkward lumbering down the fifty-five steps of a steep metal ladder to the belly of the ship. Glamorous Mrs. Fonseka, she noticed, "frisked up and down with no trouble at all."

She also worried about the other ship, the *Steel Vendor*. It had left three weeks earlier than the *Steel Executive*, and the two vessels were taking different routes, but somehow they were all supposed to meet in Calcutta. Charles Miriam was in charge of coordinating the rendezvous, but she had no idea when either ship would reach Calcutta. Cargo ships would dock anywhere they were needed to load or unload, and their itineraries were constantly changing. She decided to send telegrams at every port, to the *Steel Vendor* and to the motherhouse, and hoped the messages would reach the others fast enough to coordinate their arrival in Calcutta.

Mostly, though, Charles Miriam worried that she would fail at the one task she had been given during the journey: to learn Hindi. One of the Jesuit brothers came to see the sisters during their last days in Kentucky and gave them a brief introduction to the language and its unfamiliar script. No one in Mokama would be able to understand them unless they spoke Hindi, he told them, so it was imperative to learn the language if they wanted to be effective missionaries. Hindi was not so difficult, he said. It's perfectly phonetic; every word pronounced exactly like it's spelled, with none of the maddening irregularities of English. But it would take practice to hear and reproduce some of the sounds that don't exist in English.

Charles Miriam packed Hindi books with their cabin baggage, and she had planned to fill the idle hours on board with vocabulary and drills. Ann Roberta, the youngest, seemed to pick up the language effortlessly. She chatted comfortably in Hindi with little Karalyn Burton at every spare moment. Charles Miriam, however, couldn't seem to grasp the new sounds and patterns. She stared at the books, traced the letters, and repeated the words as she thought they should sound. But what she heard sounded so ugly, so strange, she thought it couldn't possibly be right. In one low moment, she took her book— bought with money donated by friends, family, students, and strangers inspired by their dedication—and threw it into the sea. "It's not for me! I'll never learn it!" she shouted. The other two sisters looked at her in horror.

As the ship approached the Strait of Gibraltar, the passengers caught sight of the North African coast at about four in the afternoon. Charles Miriam rushed the two younger sisters to finish their evening prayers early. They quickly ate supper and hurried up to the deck with everyone else. They didn't want to miss the view. The endless monotony of the Atlantic was finally over, and the famous Rock of Gibraltar would soon be in sight. They bundled up in their capes, tied waterproof bonnets over their caps, and stood on deck to get a good look at both shores. Charles Miriam was mesmerized by the twinkling lights of Tangiers. It looked like a fairyland, she thought.

Night fell, and cold pushed the rest of the passengers inside, but Charles Miriam insisted on remaining on deck. She wanted to see the famous rock. As the ship got closer to it, she could see only the vague outline of its towering bulk against the dark sky. Captain Green rewarded her persistence. He walked over, lent her his telescope, and showed her how to peer through it. She could see not only Gibraltar but also the city of Ceuta on the Spanish coast beyond it. When at last they got back to bed after their vigil, the sisters were chilled through and through. Charles Miriam closed her eyes, snug in a newfound determination.

The sisters became regulars on deck in the evenings, ready to witness the Mediterranean sunset, brilliant and brief. They waited each night for that thrilling moment when the sun "tips the horizon, makes a bow and quickly drops behind the curtain of the world." They saw the snowcapped peaks of Crete, and about two weeks after leaving New York, the ship arrived at its first port of call, Beirut.

The three nuns made plans with Father Wyss and the Fonsekas to explore the city. In the crowded, dirty byways of Beirut, they dodged little boys and big American cars—Plymouths, Dodges, DeSotos. They walked to the American Express office, where Mr. Fonseka had arranged for two 1947 Chryslers to take them to the old city of Damascus. They drove across failing wheat fields, sheep pastures, and a few terraced olive groves. When they reached the border between Lebanon and Syria, they were stopped at a checkpoint, where a guard demanded their papers, calling ahead to Damascus to make sure they had permission to cross. Charles Miriam noticed the differences on either side of the imperceptible border. In Beirut, with its cosmopolitan variety, they blended into the crowd. The streets were full of men, women, and children in every kind of clothing, including priests in their cassocks and nuns in black habits. Damascus, in comparison, felt austere. All the women were veiled, and Mrs. Fonseka—wearing trim slacks and a colorful kerchief tied around her hair—attracted constant attention from men, who stopped and stared.

The passengers returned to the ship, and Charles Miriam went back to her cabin. Beirut was her first glimpse beyond America, and she had the sudden feeling that she was seeing the world for the first time. The war had devastated this lovely old city while she had been safe teaching in Kentucky. The years of rationing and working double-time, years that seemed like hardship, were nothing compared to what had happened here. The wheat fields were barren and the shepherds were in rags. Their ship, and a Canadian cargo ship docked next to it, were unloading hundreds of tons of wheat—a humanitarian gesture in the absence of any other strategy by the former Allied powers. The British had recently announced their exit from Palestine, and as with India, they left no clear plans about the future. The British Army had begun its withdrawal from India, and thousands of troops had already left Bombay on ships headed to Cairo.

The sisters had hoped to go ashore at Jerusalem, to see the first Nazareth. They got so close. On November 13, 1947, the ship anchored outside the breakwater in Haifa, as it was loaded with cargo bound for

Djibouti. They watched the movements of the city—it seemed clean, orderly, and prosperous compared to Beirut, and they were eager to go ashore—but the captain warned them that the political situation was tense. There was a plan to partition Palestine, turning Jerusalem into a divided international city, like Berlin. The hours passed, and the ship remained in the harbor overnight. The next morning, Captain Green showed the sisters the newspapers. While they were docked, five foreigners had been killed in the city. Two weeks later, the United Nations approved a plan for the partition of Palestine. Cafés in Tel Aviv served free champagne, and the civil war began.

The ship docked next at Cairo, but here, too, the passengers were ordered to stay on board. The city was already full of British troops arriving by ship from Bombay, and their hastily made camp, without proper sanitation, caused a raging cholera epidemic that would kill more than ten thousand people in the country by December.

Finally, the ship reached Alexandria. All of the crew were ordered to get booster shots for cholera, and the passengers were permitted to go ashore, so the sisters went with Father Wyss and the Fonsekas to visit an old church in the city. On the taxi ride, Charles Miriam noticed the license plates—they were written in the numerals familiar to her, as well as the ones used in Egyptian Arabic. The group stopped at a money changer's stall in the bazaar, and while the priest and Mr. Fonseka haggled with him, Charles Miriam noticed a discrepancy in the numbers the money changer had written down and what he was now giving them. Gently, she pointed it out. He was startled. The guide and the money changer gestured to each other, and asked where she learned the language. You'd be surprised, she said.

At every port of call, the mail brought news from the motherhouse, prayers from their supporters back home, and news of the progress of the other three sisters on the *Steel Vendor*. But Mother

Ann Sebastian still had not given them any instructions about what to do when they reached India. Where would they stay? All they knew was that they were supposed to somehow meet the other sisters in Calcutta. But how would they know when the other ship had arrived?

Finally, at Port Said, Egypt, they got some news: the *Steel Vendor* had reached that same port about two weeks earlier, on November 3, and Sister Lawrencetta, the leader of the other group, left word that they expected to see them in Bombay, where they would dock briefly and then continue around the tip of India to Calcutta. But with the delays at every stop, Charles Miriam worried that this would be impossible. In the Indian Ocean ports, the cargo was loaded and unloaded entirely by hand. Each stop could take days. The *Steel Executive* wouldn't arrive in Bombay before November 30.

There was a message from Mother Ann Sebastian, too: Charles Miriam's rosary beads had been found. She must have left them in the taxi on the way to the Brooklyn Pier, and the taxi driver returned them to the monastery. She wrote a letter full of thanks that her pleas to St. Anthony had been answered. But prayers alone would do them little good in India. Charles Miriam took from her purse something much more useful: the piece of paper on which she had written down the name of her dentist's brother. She wrote to Mr. Charles O. Julian of RKO Pictures Bombay asking if he might be able to arrange to meet the ship when it arrived. And could he perhaps find an American priest in the city, someone who could arrange accommodations for the sisters in a convent for a night or two?

On November 27, 1947, Thanksgiving Day, the ship docked in Djibouti, its last port of call before crossing the Arabian Sea to the subcontinent. The passengers were served a feast: punch, turkey soup, roast turkey with dressing, canned Virginia ham with pineapple sauce, sweet corn, asparagus, mashed potatoes, mince pie, plum pudding with hard sauce, and coffee. Charles Miriam went to thank Captain Green for his thoughtfulness, but he brushed it aside. This time next year, when you are living in India, your rations might not be so plentiful, he warned her. Enjoy it while you can. They watched the stevedores loading and unloading the ships, carrying everything on their backs. They were so thin that Charles Miriam thought their limbs might snap under the weight. They were paid in loaves of bread.

The *Steel Executive* arrived in Karachi at noon on Saturday, November 29, 1947, slowing down as the city's long, narrow wharf came into view. What seemed, at a distance, to be cargo, just boxes and bundles, was in fact throbbing with life. Charles Miriam could see thousands of people huddled on the pier, refugees hoping to leave what had just become Pakistan to reach India. They had been leaving this part of Pakistan, Sindh Province, for months. There were men, women, children; some had come with carts and wagons pulled by donkeys, horses, or camels, others on foot. Barking dogs roamed among the crowds.

For centuries, Karachi had considered itself a twin to Bombay. They were both port cities, full of traders and troublemakers, rich merchant families and clever businessmen of indeterminate origin. The wealthiest Sindhis started leaving Karachi in June 1947, anticipating the horror to come. By July, they had transferred more than 200 million rupees out of Karachi to bank accounts in Bombay. The Partition violence began in Lahore, the main land border crossing between India and Pakistan. As it moved down the length of Pakistan, people began to leave by sea. By September, more than a thousand people a day were exiting through the port of Karachi.

By November, when the sisters pulled into the harbor, the violence

had reached Nawabshah, more than 150 miles away, and the refugees
were still coming. At that point, those leaving were the least prosperous,
the ones without enough prospects or connections to have gotten out
sooner. Some had walked with their bundles and had to sit or sleep
on whatever they carried with them. The *Steel Executive* pulled up
next to a steamer, which the captain told them was bound for Bombay. As the two ships edged closer, the sisters could see people jumping into the water, scrambling to the steamer and swarming up the
sides, hoping to squeeze into a place on board.

More than twelve million people were displaced during Partition.
Hindus and Sikhs, but also some Muslims with family in India, were
waiting to leave Pakistan, and there weren't enough ships to take
them there. Dhows, skips, steamers, and now big cargo ships had
been making this circuit for centuries. The vessels touched the cities
along the rim of the ocean like skipping stones, Djibouti, Aden, Karachi, Bombay. But the volume of refugee ships heading into Bombay—
along with the pent-up frustrations of wartime rationing and the
surge in food prices since independence—had overwhelmed the dockworkers. They had just gone on strike, refusing to unload any more
cargo until the government loosened its hold on rations and wages.
All the traffic heading into Bombay from Karachi had been stopped.

The longer the strike dragged on, the longer the steamer would
have to wait. And the longer the steamer waited, the more people
would take their chances with a dash across the harbor, trying their
luck as stowaways. Charles Miriam stayed for a while, taking in the
desperate scene, and then headed back to the cabin. The captain told
her that their ship, too, would be delayed. Even if they left Karachi as
scheduled, he had no idea what might happen once they reached
Bombay. While they were still docked, a telegram arrived that filled

her with relief. Her dentist's brother, Charles Julian, would meet them.

The *Steel Executive* pulled into the Bombay harbor on December 1, but there were twenty-four ships ahead of them waiting to unload their cargo. Captain Green gave Charles Miriam the bad news: they would be stuck in port for at least two weeks, so he didn't expect to reach Calcutta before January. He knew that the other group of sisters had left the States before they did and would be expecting to meet them in Calcutta by Christmas. Perhaps they should take an airplane to Calcutta?

The next day, leaving their things behind, Charles Miriam and the other sisters went ashore. They expected to see Mr. Julian, but it was his wife who was there to meet them. She explained that her husband was still in Delhi, where their children were in boarding school, and he hadn't been able to get back to Bombay in time to meet their ship. The trains, Mrs. Julian warned them, had become unreliable and dangerous and filled with ticketless travelers, most of them Partition refugees trying to get to safety. The trains were always late and crowded with people, who became easy prey for brigands. The police were more concerned with keeping order in the cities, and the railway police were far outnumbered.

Mrs. Julian arranged for them to stay in the city with the Franciscan Missionaries of Mary at their home, Villa Theresa, so they could break their journey and rest for a day or two. Food was strictly rationed, so they didn't want to impose on them for any longer than that. After this respite, Charles Miriam planned to keep her group on board for as long as it took for the cargo to be unloaded. The ship was still well stocked with provisions. They headed back to collect their things.

The next morning they went to the villa, walking through Bombay as tourists with the two priests. They admired India Gate, the stone archway framing the harbor of Bombay, the same spot where King George V, emperor of India, had arrived almost exactly thirty-six years earlier, making a grand entrance to assert his dominion. The last British troops made their ceremonial retreat from the same spot. Father Holland took pictures of the sisters, with the gate and a few roaming cows in the background, and they dropped off the film at a Kodak shop nearby. Charles Miriam figured they would be in Bombay a couple of weeks at least, so there should be plenty of time to pick up the prints and send them back to Kentucky to amuse their friends. Bombay, she quickly found, was a small haven of Americana. The stores and shops were stocked almost exclusively with American-made goods—Skrip ink and Sheaffer pens, and last year's vintage of Christmas cards. The British had all but disappeared.

They arrived at the villa and were greeted by the mother superior, a nun from Ireland. The Irish sisters were among the few Europeans remaining in India. Many of the Italian and German nuns had been detained as enemy aliens during the war and left as quickly as they were able to. The sisters had a light lunch—plantains, sweet limes, and tangerines—and retired for a nap to sleep off the journey.

Soon afterward, Father Wyss came to see them, carrying an urgent message from Captain Green: Don't stay on the ship, he told them. The captain had no idea how long the *Steel Executive* would be stuck in the port, and their journey could be badly delayed. They might not even make it to Bihar before Christmas. He seemed so certain of this, and so forceful in his direction. Impulsively, Charles Miriam agreed. She decided that they would go immediately with Father Wyss to change their tickets. She talked to the shipping agent for the Isthmian Lines and got a refund for the last leg of their sea voyage from

Bombay to Calcutta—$150, just enough to pay for three train tickets on the Calcutta Mail. She forgot all about the film left at the Kodak shop, told the two younger nuns to pack up, and asked the ship to send the rest of their bags—twenty-nine pieces—straight to the train station. Their journey across India was about to begin.

SIX

"Millions Are Moving and Stirring"

O ne of the oldest and longest train routes in India, the Calcutta Mail draped itself across the subcontinent like the end
of a sari. Its path stretched for more than a thousand miles
from the curve of Bombay harbor on the western coast to the holy city
of Allahabad, at the junction of two sacred rivers, and then southwest
toward the Ganges delta at Calcutta.

It was a small miracle that the Calcutta Mail was running at all.
For months, the Indian Railways had been in a state of confusion.
They had been utterly spent by World War II, when they were the
primary means of moving troops and matériel, especially the coal
that served as fuel throughout the subcontinent. They ran almost
constantly, but during the height of the war, 1942 and 1943, there
weren't enough railway cars to carry what was produced from the
coalfields of Bengal and Bihar. Those two states needed 2,800 to
3,000 railway wagons a day; at most they received 2,500. By the end
of 1943, coal output had dropped, so there were more rail wagons

available, but by that point, the railways' own stock of coal, the fuel on which the trains also relied, was running out.

The only way to keep running the coal-powered factories that produced railcars and other goods crucial to the war effort was to sharply cut back on passenger trains. Coal and railcars had been requisitioned for the troops, and when the coal ran out, the forests were cut down to make more. If the subcontinent was a body, then the thick forests of central India would be its heart and its lungs. The forests were rich with timber, coal, and minerals, but the war effort had depleted them in every possible way. The forests were burned down, incinerated for coal or sawed and split into lumber to build railway cars. In 1943, India's forests produced 863,000 tons of timber—three times the amount just two years earlier. But there weren't enough people or coal to run the railcar factories. And then there weren't enough railcars to take the coal to the troops, and not enough coal to run the passenger cars, when there were railcars available for passengers. Winston Churchill's colonial government identified this as "the mutually reinforcing problem of coal and railways."

It wasn't just coal and railways, though. The pressure on India's forests was a problem for people, too. Those who lived in the central Indian forests were encouraged to clear-cut the land, to grow food for British people cut off from other supplies. Once the British government had decided that the people of England must have not only enough to eat but weeks of food held in reserve for them, the war effort soaked up every last grain of wheat and rice that India could produce. Wheat all but disappeared from many local shops, prices rose, and Indians needed to earn cash just to eat, so they left their villages and towns to find jobs and food.

But with the trains commandeered by the army, it became harder for Indians to travel and for India's local administrators to move the food they did have from the central growing areas to the hinterlands. Churchill's wartime government refused to address this increasingly severe supply-chain problem, ignoring the countless warnings sent by colonial administrators. The resulting famine cut through the population like a scythe. Among the most consistent images in the accounts of soldiers in India during World War II is the sight of starving families. One of them wrote a letter home describing the scene from a train window on the way from Cochin to Bombay: "We could see hundreds of men, women and children of all ages on the sides of the roads and crying for alms. The sight of those half-naked wretches reduced to skeletons was too strong even for the most strong-hearted persons." He likely did not realize how closely their hunger was linked to the very train that carried him.

When the war ended—and the troops had no need of either coal or railcars—the trains began filling up again with passengers. At the end of 1947 and during the first months of 1948, there were millions of people on the move, and the American nuns were only a few of those trying to find a place in this new nation. When India and Pakistan were born, their final shapes were still unknown. In the border areas, the boundary lines were sometimes drawn right through the middle of villages. Should Muslims move to one side and Hindus to the other? Even in the interior cities, families sometimes faced impossible choices. Hindus in Muslim-majority towns and villages and Muslims in Hindu-majority places had to decide, often with very little information, where to go. Should they remain in their homes and risk an uncertain and hostile future? Or should they abandon everything that was familiar to them and make a new home in a new country, a new state, or a new village? The lucky ones had family on the other side; others were chasing only rumors of greater safety.

The three sisters had tickets for the Calcutta Mail leaving Bombay at 8:45 in the evening on Thursday, December 4, 1947. As they left the comfort of the big American ship, their home for the previous six weeks, Charles Miriam started to feel a lurch of unease. They were about to take the Indian Railways across the country, breaking their last remaining contact with the United States, and she had no idea what lay at the end of the journey.

On the way to Victoria Terminus, she insisted on stopping to buy a wash basin. They had been warned that the ones on the train would be filthy, so the sisters spent about seventy-five cents for a basin the size of a dinner plate. They might not be able to control much else about the next few weeks, but at least they could keep up appearances.

When they reached the train station, Charles Miriam was in awe. Bombay's central railway terminal was about three times the size of Louisville's Tenth Street Station. There was a cavernous central hall so filled with people that there was hardly room to breathe. Father Wyss and Mrs. Julian helped the three nuns wedge their way through the crowds to reach the platform. Refugees were sitting, standing, and huddling around in little family groups, with bundles of their salvaged belongings in the middle of each one. There were no officials in brass buttons to take care of anyone. If Mrs. Julian had not been with them, Charles Miriam thought to herself, she might not have had the courage to go inside.

In the fall of 1947, the "refugee specials" were the only trains operating. Despite the thousands of people hopping on without tickets, these trains were the only practical way to travel long distances between the cities and towns of the subcontinent. With so many vulnerable people on the move, violence on the trains became epidemic.

Militias and gangs operated with impunity. There were random stabbings, bomb blasts, and revenge killings. A railway official on the line that stretched from Delhi across to Bihar wrote, "The frequency, callousness and daring of these killings on trains and at stations has made staff very panicky and on occasions it was with difficulty that we could keep them at their posts and keep trains going." His daily reports made grim reading. People traveling on overnight passenger trains ran the risk of being murdered in their berths or thrown from the train. One man reported to railway officials that his two servants were missing. Upon investigation, the guards found their compartment filled with blood and their bodies on the tracks.

Some families decided not to risk traveling. Eddie Rodericks, the manager of the Bombay port where the *Steel Executive* had docked, for example, had a brother, Johnny, who also worked for the British administration, in the Post and Telegraph Office. Johnny was considered a rising star, so his bosses sent him to Karachi, the biggest city in Sindh. When the boundary lines were drawn and his brother ended up on the other side, in Pakistan, Eddie begged him to come home to Bombay. But his brother had a good job, his children were going to excellent schools, and Bombay was really just a short hop away on steamer ship. Why leave when the trains were impossible? He figured they would eventually be able to go back and forth to Bombay as often as they wanted. So Johnny stayed in Pakistan and didn't see his brother for years.

In India at that time, there was often no other way to move forward except to take a risk and hope for the best. A random series of events brought the sisters onto that train—a visit to the dentist, a letter to a helpful executive, a fortuitous refund. When she stepped onto that platform in Bombay, Charles Miriam gave herself over, as so many Indians did, to the whims of chance.

The Calcutta Mail pulled into the station on the evening of December 4, and the third-class passengers threw in their bags and then leapt in to squeeze their bodies into whatever space was left. The three sisters had two reserved compartments, each one the width of the coach, with a door and a window on each side opening out to the platform. The two compartments were adjacent, but there was no way to communicate between them except from the outside. The sisters had hoped to all be together, but this was the best that Father Wyss, who found a seat elsewhere on the train, could do. Charles Miriam stepped onto the train and noticed that there were no bars on the windows—earlier waves of refugees had destroyed them. She was to berth alone, with all twenty-nine pieces of their cabin luggage from the ship; Florence Joseph and Ann Roberta would share the other compartment.

Charles Miriam locked the doors and windows as best she could. These locks, she thought, paraded under the title of safety catches, but they were "about as strong and impregnable as dress hooks." Mrs. Julian had told them not to open the door for anyone. Over the next two days and two nights, she warned, the train would stop at dozens of railway stations as they traveled from Bombay on the west coast to Calcutta on the east. At any one of them, refugees might try to force their way into the carriage.

The three nuns were apprehensive, but they managed to settle themselves in for the night. Charles Miriam huddled on the seat. She needed sleep and tried to pray, but she was too scared to close her eyes. The train lurched out of the station, moving faster than she thought trains in India could manage, and the motion lulled her into sleep.

A scream in the middle of the night woke her up. "How did you get in here? Get out! Get out!" It was Ann Roberta's voice, on the other side of the wall separating the compartments. Charles Miriam sat up in her berth, and the train lurched to a stop. She heard more calling out, more voices, more footsteps. And then the voices of the railway guards mixed with those of the two nuns. "They are under this train. I saw them go under." The voices got louder, and Charles Miriam, frozen with fear, could hear the guards moving, opening the doors to the carriage, calling out, more noise, more steps.

Charles Miriam realized that the guards had caught the man who had broken into their compartment and that Ann Roberta—the youngest of all of them—had managed to keep her head through all of it. "That is he," she said of the thief. "We are afraid, and there is another sister in there all by herself." The young sisters' concern for her broke the spell that trapped Charles Miriam in terrified silence. She found her voice and called out that she was all right.

There was a crack in the wall between the two compartments, just wide enough for the nuns to speak to each other, so they told Charles Miriam what had happened. Both of them had been asleep, but Ann Roberta, in the lower berth, woke up itching with bedbug bites. She got up, swatted them off her skin, and shook out the rough linens to get rid of them. That's when she saw him: a man inside the compartment, and another one with his leg over the window trying to follow him. She screamed at them to leave. Florence Joseph woke up to the sound and pulled the emergency cord, which she could easily reach from the upper berth.

The thieves must have jumped onto the train while it was stopped at one of the early stations, Ann Roberta explained. They began by crouching under the train and waited there until it started moving. They then climbed under the compartment until they reached the space between the carriages. From there, while the train was moving, they inched around to the windows. Standing on the step outside the door, they quietly worked on the window and the metal blind, whose safety catch was easily nudged out of place. India's railway bandits had become bold and skillful; they could work so quietly that they sometimes came into compartments, opened the door, threw out the bags, and then disappeared, leaving the traveler to discover on waking that every piece of luggage in his compartment was gone.

By the time the guards arrived, the sisters realized the men had stolen Ann Roberta's purse, and with it a rosary, a flashlight, a pen and pencil set, and a packet of unread letters from home. All their money and passports, to their great relief, were in the other compartment with Charles Miriam. Once the guards took the men into custody, the train started moving again.

The sisters waited for sleep to come. The two younger sisters said the rosary twice to calm themselves. Charles Miriam felt paralyzed, as if she were choking. She couldn't utter even a word in prayer. The best she could do was to echo in her heart the rhythmic grinding of the wheels of the train with a prayer: "Mother of God, protect, protect."

At the next station, where the train stopped at about two in the morning, the police were waiting for them. They came into the carriage with the guards and asked Sister Ann Roberta to file a complaint. Charles Miriam sent for Father Wyss, who until this point had been unaware of the drama of the previous few hours. Ann Roberta described every moment in minute detail to the police officer, with Father Wyss there to translate. When she reached the point in her story where the purse was stolen, he asked her, "How many rupees were stolen?" Ann Roberta was triumphant. "That is where I have him!" she said. All the money and passports were in the other compartment. The police officers were annoyed. "All this for nothing. Start the train."

They awoke on Saturday and spent the next day watching from

the window as the train moved across India. They had not wanted to impose on the sisters in Bombay or even Mrs. Julian to pack a lunch for them—everyone's rations were limited—so they brought a big box lunch that had been packed for them on the ship: ham, cheese, and beef sandwiches, hard-boiled eggs, crackers, oranges, apples, and lemons. They ordered hot tea and cold drinks from the diner. The train moved through fields of date palm and sugarcane. The land looked so fertile, full and healthy, hiding the deprivations of the years before.

Father Wyss came over to their compartment to hear the whole tale and tried to find the humor in the situation. He had lived in India for twenty-three years and had been visited by thieves more than once but had never caught one. What unbelievable luck! he told them. The sisters not only escaped without losing anything of great value but managed to apprehend the men who did it—on their very first night in India. After every few stations, the guards would change, and with each new roster, Father Wyss would ask them, Have you ever caught a thief? No, they never had. Charles Miriam did not see the humor or her good fortune, but she later understood it to be just that— particularly after hearing of an episode in which three nurses were traveling and found thieves in the compartment. When one of them tried to pull the emergency cord, they stabbed her and tossed her body from the train.

Father Wyss tried to reassure Charles Miriam, and on their second night on the train, he planned to stay in her compartment. But by the time they reached Allahabad, the ticket agent on duty was a woman, and she would not allow it. No amount of persuasion or explanation would sway her. It was her "bounden duty" to prevent such impropriety, she told them, so Charles Miriam spent another night alone as the train made the last part of its journey to Calcutta.

Unlike Bombay, where the sisters began their journey, Calcutta had been torn apart by Partition violence. By the end of 1947, the corpses had been removed from the alleyways, but it was still a traumatized city. Everything Calcutta had once been proud of—its status as the center of colonial rule, its refined sense of itself as the steward of Indian high culture and political thought—was now in question. This had been a center, too, of Christian life in India. It was home to the Anglo-Indian community of India, descendants of white colonial men and the Indian women they took as wives or mistresses. They formed a community set apart and filled Calcutta's churches on Sundays. Missionaries of every denomination ran the hospitals, schools, and orphanages.

The Calcutta Mail arrived in Howrah Station at about five in the afternoon on Saturday, December 6, three hours later than they had expected. The Little Sisters of the Poor had agreed to host them for the night, until they could catch the train to Mokama the next morning. Charles Miriam had sent a telegram ahead to Father Batson saying they would arrive at two o'clock, so they didn't expect him to be waiting for them. Father Wyss promised to help them make their way to the convent of the Little Sisters, so they busied themselves gathering up all their bags before stepping onto the platform.

But as soon as the sisters opened the door of their compartment, a man stepped up to the train. "Is this Sister Charles Miriam?"

It was Mr. Barber, a colleague of Mr. Julian's at RKO. He and his wife knew the Little Sisters convent well. They were devout Catholics, with a daughter in the novitiate and a son already a priest. Mr. Barber told them there had been some miscommunication with their hosts, who were expecting only one sister, not three, and they did not have quite enough beds. So the Barbers insisted on hosting them all for the night.

They had managed not only to arrive safely in Calcutta, but to arrive first. Charles Miriam heard from Mrs. Barber that the other group of three sisters had traveled on from Bombay to Calcutta by ship as planned—a relatively uneventful journey—and that their ship would arrive the next day. So she arranged for them to meet Lawrencetta's group at the dock. The Little Sisters hosted Lawrencetta's group; Charles Miriam's returned to the Barbers' house, where they all spent the evening singing the old Kentucky songs at the piano and prepared for the journey to Mokama—another six hours on a train that ran upstream along the Ganges, where their mission would begin. The night before they left Calcutta, Charles Miriam confided in a letter the fear and anticipation in her heart. "These millions are moving and stirring, and we do not know how it will all end."

Celine Minj was one of those millions on the move. Like the sisters, she, too, crossed India by train in those chaotic months immediately after Partition, although she made her trip alone, knowing even less about where it might end. Those who survive such a world move forward with a particular kind of deliberation. They know they must fight—not for more, or for a better place in the world, but simply to continue to exist in it.

Celine was born in 1933 in the central Indian forests, which the sisters had crossed during their journey on the Calcutta Mail, on the tribal lands of the Oraon people in Jharkhand, a region in the southern part of the vast Bihar territory. Her elegant first name, Celine, was a glimpse into the Oraon's long contact with Belgian missionaries, who arrived in the area in the nineteenth century. These men, mainly Jesuits, lost themselves in the world of the forest. They learned the Oraon language and opened schools in villages too remote for the British colonial state to take notice.

When the Oraon converted to Catholicism, they did so as a clan. Their strength was in the bonds between and within families, so these new Catholics were able to preserve the social structures that bound them to one another. The missionaries did not, in this case, appeal to the individual's connection with this new God, but to the group, telling them that Catholicism was a tradition that might strengthen the whole while keeping it intact. The missionaries gave the Oraon one priceless gift: in the nineteenth century, when the mercantile interests of the British state and the Hindu kings began to encroach on the forests, the missionaries challenged the sale of tribal lands in court and successfully established what became India's first forest act, making it extremely difficult for tribal lands ever to be sold outside the community. It turned the tribal lands of central India into a forested island—conserved, but during the famine years of World War II, fatally isolated from the rest of the country.

Celine's father, Lazarus Minj, was a teacher in a mission school in the district of Simdega. He lived at the school, six miles away through thick forest from the house where his young wife, Mariana Tigha, was expecting their first child. Each clan in the Oraon had a sympathetic animal, one they identified with and therefore did not eat or kill, though they were otherwise omnivorous. Minj is a species of fish native to the streams and rivers of those forests. Tigha is a monkey; lakra, a tiger. Others were birds or turtles. The taxonomies of caste, language, and religion that defined every other person in India did not quite fit here, so the Oraon were called "tribals"—a clumsy label for India's Indigenous people.

When Mariana was heavy with child, Lazarus developed a high fever and died, alone, at the school. He was a beloved teacher, so the families he served built a box for his body and carried it through the forest back to his parents' village. Mariana stayed with her in-laws for the burial, watching as her husband's coffin was lowered into the ground and throwing clumps of dirt into the grave while the priests said Mass. All the schools were closed that day so the priests and Lazarus's students and their parents could attend. A week later, Mariana gave birth to a child, Celine.

Mariana was at the mercy of her in-laws, and it soon became clear that they wanted nothing to do with the young widow or her baby. They wouldn't give her any real food—only the cold, starchy water left after boiling rice. She wasn't producing enough breast milk, and she started to worry that her child would starve. Mariana's mother heard what was happening, so she walked to Mariana and brought mother and baby back home to her village in Rengari.

There, too, their position was tenuous. In the social structure of the Oraon, women needed a male protector. Without her husband, Mariana would have to look to her father. But he had died years earlier, and her only brother had died of smallpox. That left Mariana's mother living on the sufferance of her eldest brother-in-law. He decided how the family's resources would be shared, and he was stingy, allocating only three tokris of rice—a handful—every day for the two women and the infant, Celine. Mariana and her mother found ways to stretch it out. Every time they received a portion of rice, they would cook it, eat a little bit, and then save the rest in a pot with some water so it would keep. They survived on a handful of rice for two or three days.

Celine would always be tiny, but she grew tough and strong and intently aware of the difference between herself and the other children in the family, the ones whose fathers and grandfathers had lived. All of them knew hunger. Simdega was so isolated from the rest of

India that any disruption in the thin web of commerce that brought rice to their village could mean weeks of depending on whatever a family had stored up or what they could gather from the forest. It wasn't the extra handfuls of rice, however, that Celine envied. She saw the other children going to school, and as soon as she could talk, she gave voice to this hunger: "I want to study."

So Mariana again found a way. She scraped together a few annas and with that money bought rice in the market. She brought it home, cooked it, and then took it back to the market to sell. She did this over and over, and with her small profit, collected the fees to send Celine to the Ursuline Convent School nearby. Mother Ignatius could see the determination of the little girl, like that of a weed stubbornly pushing through rocky soil. Celine was never first in her class; occasionally she was second, more likely third or fourth. But no one tried harder.

Celine's will to finish school sustained her through the summers. As soon as she was strong enough, she would walk next to her mother, carrying bricks in a basket on her head at construction sites. She earned three rupees a day for that backbreaking work. Together, they earned enough for the next term's tuition, books, and pencils.

In 1945, as the war ended, Celine was twelve years old and had finished seventh grade. Her ambition to be educated had begun to cause trouble for Mariana. Here she was, a young girl, neither pliable enough to be married off nor clever enough to make her way out of Simdega. Her grandmother's sister, who was working as a nurse in Calcutta—one of the thousands of women who answered the call of World War II in the big cities—heard about this difficult girl. "You send her to me," she wrote.

Mariana bought her a third-class railway ticket to Calcutta, and Celine turned up one day at Lady Dauphin Hospital looking for her great-aunt. She would have been able to recognize Celine by the mark on the back of her left hand. Most of the families that converted to Catholicism left behind the Sarna religious traditions, but some of the old ways persisted, like the naming ceremony for children and the wearing of clan tattoos. The legend is that, generations ago, a Hindu king of the region decreed that each of the major tribal groups would use tattoos so outsiders could tell them apart. Only the women were marked in this way—a man's tribal affiliation could be traced through the marks on his mother. Celine's Oraon tattoo was drawn in neat rows: four circles, a line, a wave, a line, four circles. On either side, a wave.

Her great-aunt showed her around the hospital, but then soon left Calcutta unexpectedly. Celine thought about running away, but instead managed to talk her way onto the nursing staff, helping the trained nurses with the labor of caring for the sick, injured, and malnourished millions of Calcutta. Eventually, however, the loneliness became too much for her. One of the nurses put her on a train back to Ranchi, the biggest city in the Jharkhand region, where she enrolled in high school. She got halfway through, until the administrators sent her back home for unpaid fees.

For a while, Celine simply stayed in her village, doing nothing, consumed with envy of the girls who were still in school. Then she heard about a charity group willing to pay tuition for poor children at a local school. She got to tenth grade this way, and only had to come up with enough money for books and pencils, but this, too, proved too much. Just a few months short of receiving her high school matriculation certificate, Celine was again stranded at home.

A neighbor mentioned another way out: her niece had gone to Patna, to be trained as a nurse by the missionaries at Holy Family Hospital. This time, Celine got the railway ticket herself and ran away for good. The missionaries at Holy Family took her in, so she lived with them, and then with a Carmelite order, for whom she swept and washed without complaint. A few months after she arrived in Patna, at the end of 1947, one of the priests came to see her. "There are some new sisters coming," he told her. "They are going to open a hospital. They're American."

Amid the wreckage of a decaying empire a new nation was being born—and built.

RAMACHANDRA GUHA, *INDIA AFTER GANDHI*

SEVEN

The Opening of Nazareth Hospital

T he first time that Sister Lawrencetta Veeneman walked through the empty structure near the Mokama Junction railway station, it was hard for her to imagine that it would ever become a hospital. It was shaped like the letter L, with the main building running across the northeastern edge of the property that Batson had purchased, along the wall that separated the church grounds from the railway workers' recreation area. Another, shorter section was set at a right angle to it, away from the wall. The two floors were connected by a staircase at one end, and the whole building was encased in bamboo scaffolding.

It was a shell, a series of empty rooms, and contained no tangible evidence that it was meant to be a hospital. There were no hospital beds; no medicines; no electricity; no source of running water; no doctors, nurses, or other trained staff. The order's leadership had promised the nuns who volunteered for this mission—not to mention the people back home who had donated thousands of dollars to support them—that this building would eventually become the tenth Sisters of Charity hospital, and that it would meet the standards of the other nine. The task of leading this mission fell to Lawrencetta, and she would have six months to fulfill it.

In Lawrencetta's first letter from Mokama to her mother describing the hospital, she admitted that it was not much different from the rough diagram that Batson and the other Jesuits had sketched out for the sisters before they left Kentucky. "The convent is about as I described it to you when I was at home."

The big empty structure was built in the style of a "godown"—a word of indeterminate origin, probably Malay, that had wheedled its way into nearly every vernacular language of the former British Empire. "This word is used very frequently and nothing seems to take its place," she wrote. A godown, usually translated as warehouse, is a plain, sturdy building, and in many villages in India, aside from the mud and brick huts, it might be the only built structure other than the temple. A godown is a sign of somebody's wealth: those who need one are those who have enough to store for another day, grain to sell or goods to trade. They were often partitioned into rooms of uniform size, and were endlessly adaptable.

So when Batson promised the nuns a building that could serve as a combination hospital, convent, and school, it was perhaps not surprising that he would build a very large godown. On each of the two levels, there were a series of rooms about twenty feet square, with a double-length room in the middle. This larger space became the chapel, with the ones on either side designated as six bedrooms, a dining room, and a community room. In the shorter section, set at a right angle to the main structure, there were storerooms, a stairway to the roof garden, and a big porch.

With little else to report in those first few days, Lawrencetta described in meticulous detail the flowers in the clay pots lining the crushed-brick path between the fathers' house and the convent. There were roses, chrysanthemums, poinsettias, cannas, marigolds, bougainvillea—all of them in radiant bloom thanks to the bright midday sun and the cool nights of a North Indian winter. There were no signs of the tumult of the previous twelve months in Mokama. There were no gatherings of angry men, plotting against their neighbors. There were no columns of refugees marching away from violence. There were no more retreating British and American troops, no more cholera patients wasting away in orderly rows on cots and pallets on the ground. From two windows on the upper floor, Lawrencetta could see the railway workers settling into their evening routine. They played cards, some of them in singlets as their only shirts dried on a line in the recreation yard.

Lawrencetta was fifty-one years old when she accepted the mission to India, effectively taking over leadership of the small mission at Mokama Junction from Batson, the rogue Jesuit who had chafed at every directive handed down to him from his superiors. Now that the Sisters of Charity of Nazareth had agreed to take over the mission—at the invitation of the bishop in Patna, and with the consent and approval of the bishop in Louisville—it would be up to her to turn the empty godown into a hospital.

She and the order would be responsible for raising enough money through donations and hospital fees to get it up and running and make it self-sufficient. The Jesuits kept their house on the compound, and they continued to run the school for boys and say Mass at the shrine, but the hospital building and convent became the responsibility of the nuns. Lawrencetta knew that the Jesuits would be there to help, but her goal was to get the hospital and convent running independently as soon as possible.

She could not have been more different from Batson. Where he was full of bluster and ego, Lawrencetta approached her work as a missionary first through her vow of modesty. The previous spring, when she was still in Kentucky and first learned that she had been appointed to lead the new mission to India, she immediately wrote home to share the news. But the letter began with a description of the recent rain; the blooming dogwoods, redbuds, and japonica; and her hopes for the tulips, lilacs, and lilies of the valley. Only on the second page of her letter did Lawrencetta disclose the momentous news and her crucial role: "The group has now been appointed, and I am chosen to be one of the privileged number—in fact to be in charge of the little colony of six."

Lawrencetta's prominent role in the Sisters of Charity was a source of enormous pride for the Veenemans, a once wealthy Louisville family that had fallen on hard times. Lawrencetta's grandfather had made his fortune in coal and built a grand house in downtown Louisville, filled with piano music and song. Lawrencetta, named Marie at birth, was the second oldest of twelve children. Her father died of a kidney disease in 1916 when she was twenty, two years after she joined the convent. Lawrencetta's mother drew on a small inheritance from her father, but to maintain their house and keep the younger children in Catholic school, the oldest, a son and a daughter, started working as bookkeepers, their father's profession. Only one of Lawrencetta's sisters, Blanche, ever married. The two youngest lived at home to care for their mother and the house. Lawrencetta's decision to enter the convent meant that she would never bring in any earnings to the household—but it was a source of prestige for a Catholic family to have a daughter accepted by the Sisters of Charity of Nazareth, and an entrée to the order's well-regarded schools and hospitals.

In her first postings, Lawrencetta taught music at schools in Virginia and in Massachusetts, and then came back to work at schools in Kentucky in 1931. Mother Ann Sebastian appointed Lawrencetta as a superior at the motherhouse in 1939, guiding young novitiates toward their final vows. During World War II, her siblings had been moved by the call to serve during the war, but none went overseas. Two of her brothers were rejected for service on medical grounds, and a sister worked with the USO in Washington. By 1946, all ten of the surviving Veeneman children were still living in Louisville.

When her order announced that it was going to India, Lawrencetta had a chance to fulfill her family's wartime ambitions to serve. She wrote about the mission as something she and her mother were taking on together. "Mother, God has blessed both you and me with excellent health, and this is one way we can give Him thanks." For years, she wrote at least once a month to her mother and to her unmarried sisters, Lucy and Bernadette, who took care of their mother. Although they would never visit India, she took them along with her during the decades she spent there.

Lawrencetta's task in those first few weeks was to give the sisters a sense of purpose and security in their new home. They had no real grasp of the language or connection to the people of Mokama, and they could not really begin work without their hospital equipment, which would arrive later by cargo ship: the *Steel Executive* was still slowly making its way from Bombay around the perimeter of India to Calcutta, and the goods from the *Steel Vendor* were still waiting to clear customs.

So Lawrencetta established for the six women a routine much like the one they had followed back home in Kentucky. Every order has its rule—the carefully thought-out map for each hour of the day, apportioned to work, prayer, and rest according to a community's particular charism, its spirit or philosophy. An experienced administrator, Lawrencetta made sure that the sisters in Mokama followed the same rule as those in Kentucky, heeding Mother Ann Sebastian's warnings not to take liberties just because they were away from the motherhouse. For the first few weeks, they attempted to create a replica of the life they knew. They woke at 4:50 for prayer and Mass in the chapel at 5:30. They ate porridge, eggs, toast, and coffee, along with a surprising abundance of fruit—small oranges and bananas, papayas, guavas, and melons.

They spent much of the day immersed in learning Hindi, either in classes with one of the Patna Jesuits, Father Gallagher, or studying on their own. He drilled them repeatedly, trying to help them count to a hundred and say all the Catholic prayers in Hindi, and then moved on to the standard reader—"Ali Baba and the Forty Thieves."

Their midday meal was usually broth made from a bone bought at the bazaar and goat meat. The cook added rice or vegetables to it—cauliflower, potatoes, tomatoes, lettuce, carrots, sweet potatoes, cabbage—and they ate that along with rice and dal and a meat or vegetable curry. The sisters ate well, but they could see that Mokama was depleted. There was very little being sold in the town, and few people who could afford to buy it. "No bread can be bought in Mokameh nor eggs, butter or cheese. Once a week the Fathers go to Patna and come home with large hampers and boxes of supplies," the sisters noted in their letters home to the motherhouse. Staples were still rationed, so by the end of the week, when the bread ran out, they made do with chapatis. The sisters wrote home to Kentucky often, especially in those first few months, and kept a detailed record of the mission's activities, similar to a ship's log, called the Annals.

During their evening recreation hour, before bed, the sisters read or wrote letters by lantern light. The cold in Mokama shocked them, and they were utterly unprepared for it. At midday in early January, the temperature could reach 70 degrees, but when the sun went down, it dipped into the forties. Because the building was so new, the bricks and plaster had not yet fully hardened, so they retained moisture, and the cold and damp crept into their bodies like a thief. There was no heat in the building—no fireplace or woodstove, only their blankets and their habits, which they took to wearing at night, their capes and hug-me-tights pulled over their torsos. By the time they lay in bed, the cold started inward. They felt chills and goose bumps as their bodies tried to stir and shake some heat into them. Eventually, the weight of their blankets slowly eased them into sleep.

On January 5, 1948, less than a month after the sisters landed in Mokama, Father Birney brought a young woman to their doorstep. She was tiny, not even five feet tall, her bones like those of a bird, with deep-set eyes and skin that shone like polished wood. She had been living with the Carmelites in Patna for several months and appeared to Lawrencetta to be "a good Catholic girl" who attended Mass every day, said her rosary faithfully, and wanted to work to support her mother. Her name was Celine Minj.

Celine looked at what the sisters called a hospital and was not impressed with what she saw. There was nothing, just a small hall in a building near the railway station, and a space—the dispensary— with a few boxes of medicines. But she was a step closer to the life she wanted. She remembered those precious days at school, watching the nurses who cared for the boarding students, the ones who had no trouble paying their fees. Celine wanted to be one of those striking women walking in and out of the infirmary to check on patients who were resting, the pure white cotton of their uniforms flashing as they carefully changed a dressing. Celine could see that same competence and determination in these American women in their starched white caps. There was something so meticulous in way they went about their work, the ease with which they carried their knowledge. She had decided to stay and told herself, "I am going to become a nurse."

The hospital hadn't opened yet, so Lawrencetta offered Celine a bed on the roof. She took it, and repeated Father Gallagher's suggestion that she might help the sisters with their Hindi. The sisters were using a bilingual book—English and Hindi—to learn the names of the things around them, but Celine knew she could do better. She used her English, drawing on all her hard-fought years in the classroom, to explain to Lawrencetta and the others how to describe their new world in both languages.

Almost immediately, Celine became essential to the sisters' work. When someone turned up at the dispensary with symptoms the sisters couldn't comprehend, she translated. When they received the first calls to go out into the village to deliver a baby, Celine went with them.

About three weeks after her arrival, the cargo from the *Steel Executive* finally arrived, all of it loaded onto the goods wagon that arrived at Mokama Junction. Celine watched the controlled mayhem at the railroad station as the huge boxes and crates were unloaded from the train. "The gharries"—cars and other vehicles—"were coming in and out of here all afternoon and up until about 8:30," Charles Miriam wrote.

Batson, in his element, had rallied an army of railway porters, along with all the priests, brothers, and boys from the school, to un-load the tons of cargo and march the crates to the empty hospital. There were the fifty metal hospital beds and bedside tables, almirahs, presses, electrical wiring, ceiling fans—all the furnishings for the hospital wards that Batson had purchased in Calcutta—along with all the sedatives, vitamins, antibiotics, painkillers, and sulfa drugs that they had brought on the ship. A Maytag washing machine joined the machines that had arrived earlier on the *Steel Vendor*: a refrigerator, sewing machine, large typewriter, big clock, and a plaiter for ironing the sisters' caps. The large room meant to be used as a dispensary didn't even have shelves, so they saved the packing crates and reused them. In the evening, Celine retired to her cot while Law-rencetta led the sisters to the refectory, where they gathered with the priests for wine and fruitcake to celebrate the safe arrival of all the cargo. All things considered, it was a triumph. After more than two months on the ship and several weeks docked in Bombay and Cal-cutta, only the washing machine had been badly damaged en route.

Celine spent the next four days helping Lawrencetta and the other sisters unpack. The equipment and construction material filled the rooms in the lower level of the building, which was configured a bit dif-ferently than the sisters' quarters upstairs. There were three twenty-by-twenty-foot rooms and then a room that was three times as long. The original plan was to use the smaller rooms as a reception area and as guest quarters, but Lawrencetta wanted the hospital to be as func-tional as possible. So the two youngest nuns doubled up upstairs to free up space. The small rooms downstairs then became a receiving area for patients, an examination room, and a pharmacy. The long room became the ward, lined with the new metal beds. By January 30, patients were lining up for treatment, with Celine there to help translate their complaints and worries to the sisters. Lawrencetta

began writing letters to missions, hospitals, and medical schools all
over India to find a doctor. Nazareth Hospital—they chose the name
to honor the site of the motherhouse in Kentucky—was taking shape.

On that same evening in New Delhi, Mahatma Gandhi left his quarters after a typically full day: he had offered his private devotions,
eaten a spartan meal, read the newspapers, taken a Bengali lesson,
and spent the afternoon receiving visitors. As he walked toward a
public prayer meeting, an assassin carrying a Beretta automatic and
four hundred rupees in cash in his pocket shot Gandhi three times at
point-blank range. The mission log kept by the sisters in Mokama
recorded the news the next day. "Word was received that Gandhi was
killed by assassin. No other particulars known here. Great loss to
India. Station and public buildings draped in black. No mail to-day."

For anyone close to Gandhi, the threat of violence was nothing
new. He had been holding daily prayer meetings at Birla House in
New Delhi to face the public, who were looking to him for guidance,
and also a vocal, enraged minority of people who were beginning to
despise him for having led them into a future that seemed like a form-
less morass of hatred. Shortly before he was killed, there had been an
incident of violence against Muslims in Mehrauli, a village near
Delhi, at a Sufi shrine beloved by both Hindus and Muslims. In response, Gandhi began another prolonged fast. He was upset by the
violence and the displacement of refugees, but also by the new government's decision to withhold from Pakistan its share of Britain's
war debt, the sterling balance owed to India by the imperial government for the cost of waging World War II.

Traumatized Indians were enraged that Gandhi would presume to
fast on behalf of Pakistan when they, too, were suffering. In the weeks

before his assassination, the threats escalated and the anger came right to his door. At one point, "a batch of angry men arrived on bicycles at Birla House" shouting anti-Gandhi slogans on behalf of refugees without "food, homes, clothes and jobs." The government relented on the question of the war debt. Eventually, all the conditions that Gandhi had stipulated for the safety of Muslims in Mehrauli were met, and he broke his fast on January 18 with a glass of sweetened lime juice. But the threats continued, and two days later police found a bomb planted near the servants' quarters at Birla House by a Hindu refugee who had lost his home and said he was opposed to "Gandhi's peace campaign." There was a palpable sense that the whole country would soon be responsible for the death of their father.

Gandhi was becoming disenchanted with India's new politics. His two closest advisers, Jawaharlal Nehru and Vallabhbhai Patel, the leaders of the Congress Party, were absorbed in the task of hammering together the framework for a nation-state. Patel built India's administrative structure—he had convinced dozens of tiny former kingdoms to join the union. Nehru, meanwhile, became a roving statesman. He went to Amritsar, near the northwestern border with Pakistan, to condemn an incident in which angry refugees had trampled the flag—the new flag of independent India. Surely, he argued, the ideals that had brought them to freedom meant more than this?

After Gandhi's death, among the thousands of tributes was a private letter written by the constitutional scholar and Dalit leader B. R. Ambedkar to the woman whom he would later marry. Ambedkar, who had been raised in the community then called "untouchables," had complicated feelings about Gandhi, who he thought was beholden to caste-conscious, conservative Hindus. But Ambedkar walked for a time with the funeral procession and later wrote, "As the Bible says that something good cometh out of evil, so also I think that good will come out of the death of Mr. Gandhi. He will release people from bondage to superman, it will make them think for themselves and it will compel them to stand on their own merits." Although there would soon be other great figures towering over India—Nehru and Ambedkar among them—the new nation would have to rebuild without a superman to guide them.

About two weeks later, on February 12, India declared a public holiday for the distribution of Gandhi's ashes. The governors of each province had received a portion of Gandhi's cremated remains, which they were instructed to immerse in the Ganges or one of its tributaries, or any nearby body of water in a "grand coordinated ceremony."

While the authorities in Patna conducted the ceremony for Gandhi in Bihar's capital, the people of Mokama gathered at the railway station. "All morning there has been much activity in the recreation grounds behind the hospital," the Annals noted. "The people are being served a dinner that has been in preparation for hours. At five there was a gathering and many speakers. Fr. Gallagher was one of the speakers. At 5:10 everyone stood in silence as a tribute to Gandhi."

This symbolic effort to unite India in mourning had an obvious purpose. Many feared that, without Gandhi's moral force to bind it together, India might soon disintegrate. As one British former civil servant wondered, "What would become of the forty million Muslims left in India, who had lost their chief protector?" Nehru and Patel tried to forge a government of national unity under the umbrella of the Congress Party. And, at the same time, India began writing its constitution. The Constituent Assembly, which had been convened at the moment of independence as the de facto government of India, with representatives from dozens of India's different ethnic, religious, and linguistic groups, gathered to draft the constitution in a public process that would eventually take more than two years. It was a remarkable gesture of hope for a country that had been through so much trauma.

It was up to Lawrencetta to decide in those first few months how the order would make its way in India. The sisters' first impulse was to throw themselves into hospital work, using whatever they had on hand. Almost from the moment they arrived in Mokama, when they were still unpacking trunks, people began coming to the door asking for help. The sisters began with the medicines that Crescentia had packed in her luggage.

After the goods train arrived with their cargo from the ship, the sisters opened the dispensary every day from 10:00 to 11:30 in the morning. They weren't quite ready to open the hospital, but they wouldn't turn anyone away. A man and his wife, already in labor, arrived via tum-tum, the pony carts that were ubiquitous in Mokama. There was little the nuns could do for the woman except to boil water and ease her through the delivery. They baptized the baby Joseph, and he left the next day with his mother in a makeshift ambulance—a cane chair suspended from a stout pole carried between two men.

With their crates of medicines and nursing skills, the sisters managed to do in a few weeks what had taken Batson years: establish a direct connection with the people of Mokama. Unlike Batson, they didn't need catechists as intercessors, and they didn't keep track of the number of people they had brought into the fold. Instead, they hoped that their good work would somehow stay with everyone they treated, perhaps enough that Joseph or his parents might someday return, out of curiosity or goodwill, to learn more.

As crucial as the Jesuits were to the order's beginning in India,

Lawrencetta did not want to be under their thumb. She knew that the sisters depended on them for everything in Mokama—their weekly supplies, transport, and negotiating with the people around them, especially the men of Mokama. But when the Jesuits asked the sisters to help teach in the high school for boys, which conducted its classes in English, Lawrencetta chafed at the idea. They had not come all the way from Kentucky just to help the Jesuits with what they were already doing in Mokama. The Sisters of Charity had always run their own schools, and they wanted to start a school in Hindi, to reach as many children as possible. Feeling obliged to Batson, though, Lawrencetta reluctantly agreed. In the end, in that season of uncertainty after Gandhi's death, most of the boys did not return to school after the winter holidays. Lawrencetta was relieved. "So the school that we hope to open will be OUR SCHOOL and not a parochial school," she wrote.

Slowly, Lawrencetta figured out ways to help the sisters become more independent. She sent them on regular trips to Patna so they could see how the sisters at Holy Family ran their hospital, one of the biggest in the city. At the end of February, Lawrencetta made her own trip to Kanpur, an industrial city about 350 miles upstream from Patna in the neighboring state of Uttar Pradesh. She arranged to go by train with Mother Ingrid, leader of the Irish sisters based in Patna, so she could get bedding for the hospital from Kanpur's cotton and woolen mills. "Since there is still a ban on sending goods from one province to another, we brought back with us all our purchases—20 blankets, 200 yards of sheeting, half a dozen spreads, some ticking and table linen," she wrote in a letter to the motherhouse. There were no mills or clothing factories in Bihar, so the only way to bring those goods to Bihar was by train.

There was another reason for the trip. "Most of all I was anxious to see how the Sisters make their way around at the stations. Some of the Fathers have always been around to find us a place on the trains and we know we will not have this always." But on this trip, she gained the confidence to make her way through a railway station herself, methodically breaking down the steps in the description to her family. "When a train comes in at the station, you have to go all the way up and down to see where there is a vacancy. If there is no private place, then you have to go in with somebody else. There are first, second and third class passengers. We always travel second, and if you cannot get into the ladies' compartment, then go in first class and pay the increase if necessary."

By their first Easter in Mokama, Lawrencetta and the sisters had settled into their roles. Crescentia was the warden of the dispensary with its precious medicines. Florence Joseph was the head nurse, bustling about with the patients who came in for treatment. Ann Cornelius, "as quietly as ever," took charge of the chapel, making sure everything was in order and ready for prayers at the proper time. Charles Miriam handled the kitchen and the housekeeping, including the arduous weekly process of running the now-repaired Maytag washer. Ann Roberta became the favorite of the staff and the children on the grounds, chatting with everyone in her rapidly improving Hindi. And Lawrencetta was the one to make the "200-yard dash" across the length of the veranda to the entrance of the convent, to greet the regular stream of visitors and workmen looking for the person in charge.

After all the hours of memorizing and diligent studying, however, Lawrencetta and the others could still speak only a line or two of Hindi in conversation. The sisters could say their prayers—the Hail Mary and Salve Regina—in Hindi, although not much else. Florence

Joseph wrote to the motherhouse that the inevitable response when she tried to speak was, usually, "I don't understand."

The longer they were in Mokama, the more closely they observed the life of the town around them, and the more acutely they felt their ignorance. Crescentia grasped the hardship and suffering in front of her, but she could not cross the wall of incomprehension to know more. The experience of life in Mokama felt simple and flattened. "It's fairly easy to memorize a list of questions and orders but when the answers come, there's the catch, we often understand not a single word," Crescentia wrote in a letter to the motherhouse. When the leaves began to drop in March, for example, she noticed that people picked them up and sold them in baskets for fuel. "Who rakes up the leaves? I don't think any of us know. The 'who does what and how' is a major problem and will be till we have a better grasp on the language." Lawrencetta realized that unless the sisters improved their Hindi, the order would never fulfill its vision for what the mission could be.

Batson and Father Gallagher urged her to take the sisters to Darjeeling, where the Jesuits had a villa, during the hot season in May and June. Gallagher planned to move the language school there temporarily, so the sisters could use that time to focus on improving their Hindi. The fathers warned them not to make the same mistake they did: moving too quickly into the field before they had mastered the language. But it was hard for Lawrencetta to accept this advice. It went against her need to be out in the world, and it meant that the mission would go through still more weeks only spending money and not contributing anything to its own maintenance in the form of school fees or hospital bills. That was always their principle of operations—the order's missions were meant to be self-sustaining.

When Batson had first suggested going up to the hills, the sisters dismissed it as another one of his follies. "That amused us for we had no idea of anything like that," the Annals noted. "We thought that we just stayed here and took it all." One day of vacation a year was the norm for the Sisters of Charity, along with a brief annual spiritual retreat held close to the motherhouse in Kentucky. How would she justify the expense to Mother Ann Sebastian? The house in Darjeeling was empty—they would have to bring bedding, food, and all the supplies they might need, not to mention the cost of transporting all that luggage by train to the hills and, when the tracks ended, by car and porter up into the Himalayan foothills.

In fact, all the Catholic missionaries in the area were already making arrangements for their summer retreats. The Jesuits urged the sisters to do the same, warning them that without a few weeks of respite from the heat, they were likely to fall ill and then be of little use to anyone in Mokama.

As the hot season began, the temperature climbed quickly during the day, stirring up the hot winds and the dust storms that often follow them. The sisters tried to keep the paths sprinkled with water to keep the dust under control, but it was a tedious task that consumed vast amounts of scarce water. One day, the temperature read 114 on the veranda, and the women were starting to wither under the relentless heat. "It is the black bonnet that is a morale-breaker," as Crescentia observed.

Lawrencetta decided to accept the Jesuits' offer of two months' retreat at their villa in Darjeeling. She justified it in her letters as a way for them to complete their language study and survive the worst of the heat so that the sisters would be fully rested by the time the hospital officially opened. "We can make our retreat while at the villa, and have the formal opening of the hospital after our return. By that time we hope to have a doctor."

Their trip to Darjeeling involved a long train journey to Calcutta, then into the hills at Siliguri, where they traveled first by road and then the last three hundred feet to the villa on foot. Groups of women helped carry their boxes up the hill. Lawrencetta started to get a sense of India outside Bihar. She was struck by the clouds, watching them roll off the Himalayas as if watching "the tide on the seashore." The other sisters were thrilled by the novelty of Darjeeling after months in Mokama—the cool air, the modern open-air market full of fruits and vegetables, and "an abundance of water tumbling down crystal clear off the mountain side above us and piped into the house to every room." It was a reminder to them that not all of India was as desperate as Mokama seemed to be, and that there was nothing inevitable about the poverty and illness around them.

During their stay in the hills, they got a two-week course in Indian history and in the afternoons a double period of Hindi. Father Gallagher tried a new method of teaching. Instead of memorizing questions or lists of words, he taught them to express themselves in three-word phrases. "We want rice." "He went home." "She looks tired." They focused on speaking fluently, if simply, and the hidden world of language around them began to crack open.

Celine, too, came with them. She and Lawrencetta had formed a close bond during those intense first months, and Celine became Lawrencetta's constant companion. On Lawrencetta's birthday in February, Celine brought her six duck eggs on a plate lined with marigold petals, along with a card she drew and decorated.

On one of those temperate days in Darjeeling, Celine took up her pen and wrote to Mother Ann Sebastian herself. While Lawrencetta was learning Hindi, Celine was getting more confident every day in English. After starving as an infant, enduring years of deprivation to learn the secrets of books and numbers, and surviving hundreds of miles of perilous train journeys on her own, she had finally reached the point where she could speak for herself and announce her own desires. "Good day to you," she wrote. "I am Celine Minj, who lives with The Sisters of Charity, Nazareth Convent in Mokameh. I help them if I could. Mokameh is a very beautiful place. I like it too much." Celine had seen the world outside the forests of Jharkhand and wanted to be fully part of it. She was stunned by the cold of the hills in Darjeeling and the mist that shrouded them, and she thrilled at the memory of the trees heavy with mangoes in Mokama. "Oh Mother, if I say mango then comes out water with my mouth, really Mother."

Lawrencetta and the other sisters used their time in the hills to write letters to check on the progress of repairs and renovations at the hospital, including partitions dividing the space further so there would be a few private rooms, an operating room, and a delivery room. They also replied to the messages from their supporters in the United States, gently insisting that they did not need magazine subscriptions and that most donations of household goods might not be worth the import duties to send. What they needed was money and, of course, a doctor of their own. Lawrencetta asked for prayers, wrote letters, and placed advertisements in English-language newspapers for Catholics in southern India. Madras Medical College, the best in the country, was in the south, and they hoped to find a doctor that way.

By the time the sisters returned to Mokama, it was again time for planting. The sisters had survived the cold, the dust, and the heat, and the monsoon had begun. Lawrencetta's hope came through, again, in her letters. Everything was green, and she had seen corn growing more than a foot tall. She reported back to her family about the progress of the seeds they had sent her. "We have a nice plot for a garden, and I lost no time in getting the seeds planted, which Henry gave me," she wrote. "It is true they are last year's seeds and may not be good, then the ground is not very rich, and this may not be the proper time here for planting many of these, but I thought I would take a chance rather than throw the seeds away." The hospital building was ready, its floors swept clean with brooms procured from the departing American troops. There was a shortage of kerosene, so they used it as sparingly as possible, and Lawrencetta wrote her letters quickly before dark. The opening date was set for July 19, she wrote. "Please redouble your prayers that we will get a doctor by that time."

EIGHT

"He Is Young, Energetic and Enthusiastic"

O n July 24, 1948, a Saturday morning just days after the opening of Nazareth Hospital, a young man walked into the mission while the sisters were gathered for morning Mass. Lean, strong, and quiet, with thick hair that he kept combed in a stylish wave, Dr. Eric Lazaro had arrived as promised.

He was not their first choice. The same day he accepted their offer, Lawrencetta got a letter from a woman answering the same newspaper ad. "I am only sorry that we did not get the lady doctor first, because that is what is needed most in our section of the country," Lawrencetta wrote in a letter to the motherhouse. But he was as good a substitute as they were likely to find, a capable doctor around whom they would build the rest of the staff.

Eric Lazaro was born in 1921 to an Anglo-Indian family originally from Madras. His father was a doctor, an obstetrician in Kabul, who was working there with his wife and young son. When Eric was six, his mother died, possibly of tuberculosis. He thought fondly of Kabul, the place that held his only memories of his mother. But her death destroyed their young family. His widowed father drank heavily and, unable to care for Eric, sent him back to Madras, more than a thousand miles away on the southeastern coast of India, to live with his Aunt Stella, who had a house close to the beach. They sent him to St. Bede's, his father's old school—one day Eric found the familiar name scratched into a desk—but he never quite belonged, knowing that he had been abandoned by his father and was there only on the forbearance of his relatives.

As soon as he finished high school, Eric started medical school, scraping together just enough money to pay his fees. He didn't always have enough left over for food, but he was kind and open and always had friends, so he would sit with them in the dining hall and eat their leftovers whenever he was short. He was fast, too, and he raced at a track where people bet on the runners. When exam time came around and he needed a suit to sit for them—Madras Medical College followed the English rules of decorum for students—he would race, collect his winnings, buy a suit just before the test, and then sell it as soon as he finished and recoup some of the money.

As his final exams and the end of medical school approached, Eric knew he would have to find a position on his own; he couldn't expect his relatives to continue supporting him once he was a doctor. He was among those millions set adrift in that uncertain period after the end of the war but before independence, but unlike many of his classmates, Eric Lazaro would not be able to lean on family connections to find his way. He was on his own. Eric had friends who were working at the prestigious Catholic hospital in Patna, and he heard about the new American hospital about to open in Mokama. It was a nowhere town, but he was a doctor with no experience. The nuns would provide room and board, and he was ready to leave everything else behind.

Eric's estrangement from his family proved to be his most important qualification. He was willing to dedicate himself completely to the work of Mokama, to be the only doctor for a hospital serving tens of thousands of people. There were very few other trained physicians in India who were willing to do that or to work in such a place. The sisters didn't have separate quarters for him, so he slept in the doctor's office downstairs, showered in the priests' house on the other side of the compound, and took all his meals with the sisters. Lawrencetta noticed that his initial shyness seemed to lift. "He is young, energetic and enthusiastic," Lawrencetta wrote to her family. And in Nazareth Hospital, he found a home.

The difficulty of finding doctors in India was not limited to Mokama. Just a few years earlier, in the darkest days of World War II, the shortage of doctors was, in fact, a subject of intense concern to British authorities. In October 1943, in the midst of a severe famine, the colonial government of India sent a letter commissioning a "broad survey" of health conditions, medical facilities, and institutions in British India to make recommendations for "future development" after the war was over. There had never been a comprehensive survey of the state of India's health before, and the commission knew that, with the wartime restrictions on travel in place and so much of the colonial administration devoted to the war effort, it might be difficult to do the detailed, on-the-ground research that was needed. Nevertheless, the committee was encouraged to "plan boldly."

The health survey could have turned into one of those grand colonial projects that accomplished little except to reveal Britain's imperial overreach. In the nineteenth century, for example, colonial administrators used the census to classify India's castes, taking a malleable and extraordinarily complex social system and simplifying it into fixed categories that reflected racist assumptions. But the health survey was placed in the hands of Sir Joseph Bhore, a distinguished Indian bureaucrat who brought to the commission a dedication forged during decades of devotion to public service. It was the most significant assignment of his life.

Born into an Indian Christian family, Bhore served for years as the diwan, or chief adviser, to the maharaja of Cochin. He married a missionary doctor, Margaret Wilkie Stott, and later was posted to London and then New Delhi, where he was appointed a member of the viceroy's executive council in 1929. Bhore served the Crown loyally, even as Gandhi's independence movement gathered force, and he retired with a knighthood in 1935 to the island of Guernsey. Bhore was forced out of his quiet retirement when German forces occupied Guernsey and the other Channel Islands in 1940. He lost his property, and with nowhere else to go, he went back to India.

Bhore took his mandate seriously, recruiting more than two dozen British and Indian doctors and colonial public health officials to serve on his committee and dispatching them to every corner of India. The Goodenough Committee had conducted a similar survey for Great Britain, but in the same amount of time, about twenty-six months, Bhore's committee had covered not only a much wider territory— they managed to visit every province in British India except Assam and Baluchistan—but also a wider range of inquiry, from patterns of mortality to the status of health education and professional medical training. The committee compiled detailed nationwide statistics on the prevalence of serious diseases, including malaria, dysentery, cholera, and other waterborne diseases and descriptions of social practices, including child marriage, that were particularly harmful to the health of women and children.

The result, which has become known as the Bhore Committee Report, is a startlingly bleak picture of what it meant, physically, to be an Indian at the time of independence. The starkest numbers were among children. The first ten years of life for Indians were incredibly treacherous. In 1941, of every 1,000 babies born, 158 would not survive their first year. Children under ten accounted for nearly half of all the deaths in India every year. The huge number of deaths at young ages depressed the overall figures for life expectancy, which stood at only twenty-seven for men and women in India. The life expectancy numbers "tell the same tale" as the child mortality figures, the report explains, "because they express in terms of the probable length of life of the individual the cumulative effect of the specific mortality rates at different ages." Death, in other words, stalked the children of India mercilessly.

But what comes through in more than a thousand pages of detail is Bhore's essential optimism for India, even at a time when nothing about the country's future was certain. He had presented, in heartbreaking detail, the toll that hundreds of years of colonial neglect had taken on the bodies of hundreds of millions of Indian people, and yet he believed, in his technocratic way, that Indians themselves could reverse the effects of generations of cruelty. Bhore's report presented a concrete plan for what India should do and what it would cost.

The overall goal was simply to increase the number of doctors and other health professionals. There were far too few to serve the size of the population—only 1 doctor for every 6,300 people in India, compared to 1 for 1,000 in England. Bhore set a target of increasing the ratio to 1 for 2,000 by 1971, an expansion comparable to what Russia had achieved in less than thirty years. In 1945, the government of India was spending only 3 annas per person ($^3/_{16}$ of one rupee) on health. He proposed raising that to about 1 rupee, 3 annas during the first five years after independence, and doubling that in the subsequent five years.

The report imagined a network of small village health centers: a trained doctor would be in charge of several villages, serving a population of about twenty thousand with a staff of thirty-eight people. "A lady doctor will also work in this group of villages when sufficient women are trained as doctors." Each small village center would include a dispensary and five-bed emergency unit. For every three centers, there would be a thirty-bed hospital, as well as two doctors, two nurses, four midwives, and four traditional birth attendants who go out for deliveries. He imagined that these units would start in some parts of a district and extend over an entire district as more people were trained.

Bhore felt strongly that ordinary people, not just trained professionals, would have to be involved. Each center would have a "health committee" of "enthusiastic village workers" who would work in their own communities on general public health education and sanitation. "Without this goodwill, the Health Committee are of the opinion that these schemes will not succeed." Above the primary centers, he proposed secondary health centers serving a population of six hundred thousand, with specialist staff and lab facilities, and beyond that a district hospital with two hundred beds and "medical and surgical aid of a high order."

This was one of the very few moments when someone in the government of India saw with absolute clarity what was required to change India for the better. Bhore believed that India's vast population, dispersed across millions of villages, need not be an obstacle to change. Its people could be made part of it. The report recommended that the primary and secondary care centers be left to act independently and work with their communities to deal with the most pressing health needs. The report was greeted with fanfare. *The Times of*

India trumpeted its release on December 27, 1945: "For the first time in the history of India, a comprehensive plan for health." But within a year, as its proposals were overtaken by the more urgent political challenges of Partition, Bhore's ambitious vision of India faded from view. If the women of Nazareth read or took notice of the Bhore Report before they agreed to take on the Mokama Mission, there is no sign of it in their records.

As soon as the hospital opened officially, patients began coming every day, a stream of people from Mokama and the surrounding villages with cholera and malaria and unspecified fevers, men with infected wounds, and women in labor. The mission Annals and the sisters' letters home, which were at first so full of homesickness for Kentucky—Lawrencetta would sometimes weep while reading letters from the motherhouse—were instead occupied with detailed accounts of the people who streamed into the hospital, what the sisters were able to do for them, whether they lived or died, and the occasional novelty of a wealthy patient who arrived by motorcar or summoned a doctor and nurse for a house call made by elephant.

The supply of medicines and equipment they brought with them as cargo—antibiotics, penicillin, painkillers, bandages, disinfectants—were usually enough to treat the most common illnesses and injuries. But occasionally they could do little but act as witnesses, for the woman in the throes of a psychotic episode or the baby in the final stages of dehydration.

Dr. Lazaro proved himself to be an able and resourceful doctor and part of the community. In addition to treating the constant stream of infections and tropical diseases, he helped with eye surgeries at a temporary clinic set up by some visiting doctors. He did the autopsy for a beloved orphan boy who had lived at the convent for months but eventually died, his enlarged spleen revealing the toll of malaria and kala-azar, a disease spread by sand flies. He managed to operate on a woman with an ectopic pregnancy by lantern and flashlight, and with the help of a visiting surgeon, he operated on Sister Florence Joseph when she had appendicitis. And when one of the servants, Doma, who had come back with them from Darjeeling, decided to be baptized, Dr. Lazaro served as her godfather.

The days passed quickly. After escaping the punishing dry heat of high summer, the sisters opened the hospital during the enveloping monsoon torpor of late July and August. It was so humid that even without much rain they were soaking wet all the time. It took days for clothes to dry, and flies tormented them at the table, descending over their plates and teacups. There were so many patients, however, that they hardly noticed these inconveniences. In August, the sisters began recording their census of patients: nineteen in the hospital and sixty-one in the dispensary on August 7. By the end of that month, both were overflowing.

Once the hospital was running, the sisters adjusted their roles, with Ann Cornelius and Florence Joseph taking on much more responsibility as the nurses in charge of the hospital, and Crescentia fully occupied with the dispensary. Patients filled the hours between dawn and dusk, and Lawrencetta had to adapt their evening routine into a streamlined version of the "rule of hours" at the motherhouse: Rosary at 5:35 p.m., supper at 6:00, spiritual reading at 7:15, and recreation from 7:35 p.m. to 8:30, before evening prayers and lights out at 9:30.

That hour of recreation was a jealously guarded time. It was when the sisters wrote to their families, played cards, and told one another stories about the amusing people and baffling or difficult cases they encountered each day. They were often so busy that they might go through the whole day without time for a real conversation. There was very little kerosene available in Mokama and no electricity in the hospital, so they tried to eat their meals while there was still daylight and use the lanterns sparingly. At night, they learned to sleep despite "the jackals' serenades, which sound like women in great agony."

The sisters took advantage of the two months of pleasant weather—October and November—to again reconfigure the rooms on the bottom floor of the building and make other improvements. They added windows all around the ward, "making it very light and airy." They added a partition to one side of the operating room to separate an area for the sterilizer and the scrub room. Those empty rooms of the original godown had become, in order, a doctor's office, the dispensary's treatment room, a pharmacy, the C ward for women, the B ward for women, a combination chart room/linen room, then the A ward for men, a nursery for children, two isolation wards for tuberculosis patients, the doctor's bedroom, one private room for wealthy patients, the delivery room, and the operating room. They moved the presses out of the dispensary and added a door from the toilet room to the veranda on the outside for the doctor, who no longer would have to go to the priests' house for his shower. The lack of running water did not prove to be a serious obstacle: Crescentia set up a still to produce purified water, a jury-rigged contraption that Charles Miriam quipped would not be out of place in the hills around Nelson County, Kentucky. By the end of 1948, a year after they arrived in India, the sisters had grown more confident in their work. They celebrated the first anniversary of their arrival by establishing a mobile dispensary in Aunta, a village about ten miles away. With their medicines packed in cases, Dr. Lazaro, Charles Miriam, and Crescentia

went out to the village twice a week, receiving patients on the veranda
of a private house.

Throughout those first few months, the sisters scrambled to find
enough nurses to help. Lawrencetta wrote a letter to the motherhouse
in September 1948 describing the scene at the hospital. "In the dispensary, during the hours that it is open, besides Sister Crescentia and
the doctor, it takes one for giving treatments, one for admitting patients and at least two others. We are finding it as difficult to get some
trained nurses as it was to get a doctor."

Here, too, Bhore had foreseen their difficulty: the committee's report included a detailed section on the status of nursing at the time. It
was hard to know precise numbers because many nurses registered
their qualifications with more than one state, but the committee estimated that there were about 7,000 nurses in all of India—one nurse
for every 43,000 people, in a country of 300 million. "There are not
in the whole of India today so many qualified nurses as there are in
London alone," the report noted.

While there were about 190 schools across India where "training
recognized by the Nursing Councils is undertaken," the standards
fell far short of those in most modern nursing schools. In fact, they
were not really schools at all. They were simply schemes under which
women would work at hospitals without pay under the title of "nurses,"
learning what they could on the job and providing free labor to hospitals in the meantime. "Furthermore, in no hospital is there a staff
adequate either in numbers or in experience to provide the necessary
instruction and the supervision of training." The report recommended
the creation of a new national body to certify those standards, and
minimum standards for classrooms and curricula.

India's nurses were almost entirely women, and the lack of formal instruction or professional accreditation, the low status of nurses, and the "deplorable" conditions in which they had to live and work were the main impediments to increasing their number. "As long as such conditions obtain it is inconceivable that Indian women from the more educated families will enter that profession in appreciable numbers."

Lawrencetta was constantly asking the hospitals in Patna, the Patna Jesuits, and other orders in Bihar to send them nurses, even those who hadn't completed their training. Holy Family Hospital in Patna sent them one or two at a time, on loan for a few weeks: Miriam and then Hilda; Rosemary and Johanna. A priest sent them two girls from Travancore, recent Catholic converts, who had some nursing training but no certificate, and a Belgian nurse who stopped at Mokama for a while on her way to Calcutta. Later, there was Miss Macqueen, "a grand nurse in every way," who spent three months in Mokama but then back went to Patna to complete her training in midwifery. There were Teresiama and Rose, and Sister Mary Kieran, a nurse from an order in Jamalpur.

The lack of clear standards for nurses in India was very obvious to the sisters at Mokama. One left for a vacation and never returned, another turned out not to be a nurse at all but a compounder, who had worked in pharmacies mixing and preparing medicines but who could not even manage to use a syringe. They sent one Holy Family nurse back after two months. The Annals noted simply: "We have not found her satisfactory."

So the sisters made do with the people they had. Florence Joseph took over the night shift. Doma, their servant from Darjeeling, helped with the patients' trays. Seraphina, one of their household staff who lived in the village next to the hospital, did the cleaning. Celine, who had been translating for the sisters and doing whatever else needed to be done, was assigned to register patients and help in the dispensary. Her crucial role in communicating between patients and the sisters was formalized, and she was a step closer to nursing. But none of these makeshift solutions was enough to deliver the standard of care that the sisters expected of themselves, Lawrencetta wrote. "Twice, our twenty-eight bed hospital has been filled with thirty-one and thirty-three patients, but we now have to draw the line and close down one of the wards until we get more help, as the Sisters are just wearing themselves out."

The new year, 1949, began with the arrival of yet another young woman hoping to help in the new hospital. Josephine "Babs" Gillard arrived on January 17. Olive skinned, with almost Polynesian features, she looked different from most of the other women who turned up in Mokama. She wore a dress, not a sari or salwar kameez, and kept her hair short in a fashionable bob. The Annals recorded her arrival with enthusiasm: she was a "marvelous help, so intelligent and so willing to do" whatever needs to be done.

Babs Gillard's family was already well known to the sisters. They lived in Calcutta, where they were active members of the small Anglo-Indian Catholic community and had often gone out of their way to help the sisters on their frequent trips to that chaotic metropolis. Anglo-Indians occupied a strange place in Indian society. They enjoyed certain advantages in the colonial bureaucracy, but they were often looked on with suspicion. Most of them wore only Western clothes and some could pass for white. Because they were Christian, they were considered outside the caste system, so they took up professions, like working with hair, that upper-caste Hindus considered polluting. Many Anglo-Indians were unsure of their place in independent India—other Indians questioned their loyalty, especially those who had served with British forces during the war—and left as soon as they could for England, Canada, or Australia.

Joe Gillard, Babs's father, worked for the railways, so the sisters called him whenever they needed help at the station. Just before Babs arrived, Mother Ann Sebastian and her successor, Mother Bertrand, came all the way from Kentucky for a whirlwind visit to see the new hospital for themselves. The sisters were keen to impress the mothers superior with their progress and make sure the visit went off smoothly, so they went to the Gillards. The family arranged for a car to take the two elderly women around Calcutta, and saw them off at the station for the journey to Mokama.

Joe was a gregarious man with a healthy sense of humor about himself. He was unusually dark skinned for an Anglo-Indian—his wife's family nearly disowned her for marrying him—and he used to call himself "Old Black Joe." His life revolved around his family, his friends, and his Church, and he joked that if there was any Anglo in him, you couldn't see it in his skin, only in his habits. He went through four packs of cigarettes and twenty rosaries every day.

Babs loved him, though. Her mother, Muriel Gillard, died when she was only four, and Joe tried his best to rebuild their life after that tragedy. He seemed to have more love in his heart than any one person could absorb. Joe remarried after his wife's death, a woman named Cookie, and adopted her children, Toots and Louie; he all but adopted his brother's children, too. Babs wasn't alone—she grew up with her stepsiblings and her cousins and called them all brothers and sisters—but nothing could fill the void left by her mother's death.

Babs had gone to St. Rita's, a fine Catholic school in Calcutta, but she left after a few years. World War II opened some possibilities:

Babs joined the Women's Auxiliary Corps (I) and served as a telephone operator, one of the many Indian women who kept communi-
cations going for the British forces when the railroads and telegraph
lines were attacked. It was glamorous, and it gave her a chance to
belong to something bigger than herself.

But at the end of the war in 1945, she was twenty-two years old, a
single Anglo-Indian woman with a fourth-grade education and no
clear idea of where she belonged. She drifted from one odd job to the
next, working as a hairdresser and a masseuse and tailoring her own
dresses. She was uneasy in Calcutta. A friend of one of her sisters had
married a British man, and Babs heard that the young woman, visibly
pregnant, had been murdered in the street during the Partition violence. Like her father, Babs felt close to the Church. She tried to join
Mother Teresa's new order in Calcutta—the Albanian nun had been
living in India for years, and started her new mission to the poor at
about the same time that the Kentucky sisters did—but they rejected
her. Finally, one of the Patna Jesuits told her about the American nuns
in Mokama who desperately needed help, and the priest arranged for
her to join them. Joe Gillard got his daughter a free railway ticket to
Mokama.

In the first few months after her arrival, Babs, too, quickly became
part of the Nazareth family. She was Crescentia's right hand in the dispensary, maneuvering her petite frame around the little room to re-
trieve the bottles of vitamins and penicillin arranged in the packing-crate
shelves. When Babs's cousin Marie required a thoracoplasty—a removal of the ribs, often done to treat a lung diseased from tuberculosis—
she traveled all the way from Calcutta to Mokama for the procedure.
It was a major surgery, so Joe Gillard arranged for ice and oxygen to
be sent by train from Calcutta, and Sister Elise, a surgeon at Holy
Family, came from Patna to perform the operation. Marie spent weeks

in the hospital afterward under Dr. Lazaro's care, with Babs at her bedside.

Even with Babs to help her, the strain and overwork eventually became too much for Sister Crescentia. On the night of March 30, 1949, she had a series of heart attacks. When she did not appear for Mass the next morning, the dachshunds she loved so much—Batson had sent them to chase away the rats that chewed through the medicine crates—were barking and yelping and trying to pull the covers off to get her to wake up. Dr. Lazaro had been trying to get her to rest. He had warned her that she was working too hard, and overexertion was dangerous when she was still taking a drug to treat dengue fever. He now ordered her to spend the rest of the hot months recuperating. He and Babs would remain at the hospital and run the dispensary while two groups of sisters went in turn for their annual retreat to Darjeeling.

Crescentia managed to make the annual trek up into the hills by train, but she was helpless. The sisters had to hire coolies to carry her in an "invalid chair" every step of the way—from her room, where the chair was loaded into a Jeep, to the train station, where the coolies were waiting to carry her straight into the compartment for the train to Calcutta. An ambulance arranged by Mr. Gillard helped her make the transfer to Darjeeling and a waiting car. For the last bit up the hill in Darjeeling, the part that was too steep for the car, porters had to carry her to bed.

The sisters were back in Nazareth Hospital by July 11, and three days later, Lawrencetta gathered them all for supper to deliver some news: Dr. Lazaro and Babs Gillard were to be married, to no one's great surprise. "This announcement came as a climax to many months' conjectures on the subject," the Annals noted. The couple intended to remain at the hospital, a relief to the sisters, who knew that the doctor could easily find a position at triple the salary they paid him. The Gillard family visited a few days later, on July 18, to celebrate Babs's birthday and her engagement. She was twenty-six.

Soon afterward, Nazareth Hospital opened its "nursing school." After Crescentia's illness and with the number of patients growing every day, Lawrencetta was convinced that they could no longer manage without a reliable source of trained nurses. They didn't have any kind of official recognition for the nursing school, but they had set aside a room and some tables and chairs, and the sisters and Dr. Lazaro taught the various subjects—anatomy and first aid, nursing arts, dietetics, and the routines of patient care.

The first students were three of the haphazardly trained nurses who had landed up in Mokama hoping to work—and Celine, whose desire and enthusiasm for nursing had never wavered. The school also accepted three Maltese sisters from Jhansi, a historic city a few hundred miles to the west of Mokama. The sisters were also trying to begin a mission hospital, and the American sisters were happy to take them in for training. The Maltese sisters preferred to chat with one another in Maltese and said their prayers in Latin and Italian, but they seemed eager to learn.

It was up to Crescentia to gain official recognition for the school. She went to Patna to see the head of the Bihar Nurses Registration Council and returned the next day "quite satisfied." The school was not recognized yet—it did not have dedicated classrooms or dormitories, one of the key recommendations of the Bhore Report—but the administrator, Miss George, promised to visit. She arrived in November and told them that the hospital was too small for the number of nurses they had taken on to qualify as adequate training. But she stayed to watch a major surgery and was impressed with their technique and standards. Once they expanded their facilities, with real nurses' quarters and classrooms, she would come back to make it official.

It is hard to overstate the boldness of what the sisters at Nazareth Hospital had accomplished. By December 1949, the sisters made a note in the Annals about all the people helping them—the doctor, four helpers in the dispensary, seven nurses, three working in the hospital, three girls in the house, a cook, two kitchen helpers, a water carrier, a night watchman, a handyman who kept the generator running inside the powerhouse, three hospital sweepers, a gardener and his helper, and the washerman and his family, who handled the endless laundry. All together there were thirty on the list. It was perhaps not exactly what Bhore had in mind when he imagined the thirty-six staff assigned to two doctors. But it was close, and the sisters had fulfilled Bhore's recommendations almost to the letter, setting up a basic primary-care hospital and village health center that devoted most of its resources to easily treated communicable diseases and infant mortality and delivery, and a new school to train nurses.

More remarkably, Nazareth Hospital was self-sufficient. The Annals recorded an income for 1949 of 109,861 rupees—a bit less than half of that from receipts at the hospital and the rest from donations. That was more than enough to cover their expenses of 92,290 rupees, which included the cost of buying their cottage retreat in Darjeeling. Lawrencetta and the other sisters had brought their vision of a working hospital to life, less than two years after they arrived.

The six sisters had every reason to be proud of that accomplishment, but the Annals of the Christmas season of 1949 devoted much more space to another event: the wedding of Dr. Lazaro and Babs Gillard, the two motherless children who had found love and a home in Mokama. The sisters insisted that the couple hold their wedding right there at the convent after the end of the Christmas holy days.

The sisters gave a wedding shower for Babs Gillard and Dr. Lazaro on the twenty-fifth, and two days later, the Gillards and their friends arrived from Calcutta. The men stayed in the priests' house, the women in the hospital. A doctor from Patna arrived to replace Lazaro during his honeymoon.

On the morning of the wedding, December 28, the sisters held their prayers in the chapel. All the kneelers had been taken to the shrine for the ceremony, so they knelt on the floor while Babs and the bridal party dressed in Sister Crescentia's sick room downstairs—she was ill again and on bed rest. There was no record of anyone from the Lazaro family attending, although the shrine was full of his and Babs's friends, including one who served as Dr. Lazaro's best man. Babs's cousin and stepsister served as the bridesmaid and flower girl.

The sisters and Dr. Lazaro all made their way to the shrine to wait for the bride. There was an awkward moment when Dr. Lazaro found himself standing at the altar and Babs was nowhere in sight. After a bit of confusion, it turned out that the driver had forgotten to go back and get her, assuming she would just walk the half mile from the convent to the shrine. But the rest of the ceremony went off beautifully. The sisters sang the High Mass, and a soloist sang one of Dr. Lazaro's favorite hymns.

Lawrencetta, in her understated way, reported the news to her family in her last letter of the year. "On Dec. 28, our medical officer, Dr. Lazaro, and Babs Gillard, who has been working at the registry desk in the dispensary, were married at the Shrine. They are devoting their lives to mission work in the hospital." Because they were both on the staff and both living there, "the reception and breakfast were held in our parlor." They had coffee and sandwiches in the morning, and for the dinner reception, the priests from the nearby town of Bar Bigha sent twenty pounds of fresh beef—then all but contraband in the area—by a messenger who carried it by bicycle in a box to hide the contents. "Quite a unique event in the history of a hospital."

NINE

Heartbreak

A patient walking to Nazareth Hospital in the early weeks of 1950 could see at a glance exactly how busy it had become, even before entering the gate. If there was a crowd gathered under the mango trees outside, there was sure to be a long wait. People began lining up to visit the dispensary as soon as it opened in the morning, and once the reception area was filled, the latecomers gathered outside.

Those who were very sick would be admitted to the hospital and placed under the care of Dr. Lazaro. He made his rounds with his new bride; Babs's Hindi was better than her husband's, since she had grown up in Calcutta, so she helped him interview patients. The sisters were endlessly grateful that they had found a couple willing to dedicate their lives to the mission of the hospital. They were impressed with the doctor's devotion—he prayed fervently to Our Lady of Fatima when the priests brought the statue to bless the operating room one day—and the couple's willingness to live at the hospital, since the sisters hadn't quite gotten around to building a proper doctor's quarters. Babs and Dr. Lazaro slept in room 2 of the hospital in a bed that Lawrencetta had given them as a wedding present.

The hospital was so busy, however, that everything and everyone involved with it was stretched to the limit. The local darzi, or tailor, was there every day making mattresses, pillowcases, new habits, aprons, and capes. "Our clothes are wearing out," the Annals noted, and the sisters bought forty new metal hospital beds to replace the folding army surplus cots that Father Batson procured for them when they first arrived.

The most dire shortage, as ever, was nurses. Two trained nurses and one pharmacist—and the rotating cast of temporary nurses—were simply not enough to care for all the patients. "Sister Florence Joseph has had to look after the operating room as well as the hospital and do all the sterilizing. She has been very much overworked."

The provisional nursing school, which began with seven students in 1949, was down to four by early 1950. The Maltese sisters, whom Lawrencetta had welcomed with high hopes, were ill-suited to the hard work and the harsh climate of Mokama, and they left with Lawrencetta's blessing. "We like the Sisters individually but they have not shown a very earnest spirit about their studies," the Annals noted. Of the remaining four nurses in training, only two, Celine Minj and Michael Gaetano, seemed prepared to take their preliminary exams. Normally, a student nurse would need her matriculation certificate from high school even to be considered for the nursing exam, but Celine was confident that with all her time in the hospital, she had absorbed more clinical knowledge in a few months than most nursing students did in years. As the sisters remarked in the Annals, "It would not have been very good for our nursing school if the first candidates went up for exams and did not pass."

Celine and Michael both passed, and the state government gave Nazareth Hospital temporary permission to continue the school, under one condition: by January 1951, the sisters would have to build more hospital space and add more beds and accommodate more patients. Without enough patients, the nurses wouldn't get adequate instruction and the school would lose its recognition.

This posed a problem for Lawrencetta. The hospital was self-sufficient at its modest initial scale, but she had no capital to expand. She wrote to the motherhouse with a formal request for money to pay for an expansion. "That is why we must have satisfactory rooms for the nurses to live and eat in and suitable classrooms," she wrote. "This we hope to accomplish by that addition going up on the north wing." The approval for expansion came from the motherhouse by cablegram on March 19. Lawrencetta was grateful. "Deo gratias and god bless Mother for her generosity," she wrote. She was also prepared. She had kept the old army cots and planned to use them as beds for the new nurses' dormitory.

To fill those beds, Lawrencetta started recruiting nursing students, which proved to be as difficult as finding trained nurses. The scarcity was especially acute in a place like Mokama, where local women rarely had formal schooling and the town was too remote to attract young, educated women from other parts of India. Lawrencetta leaned heavily on Holy Family Hospital in Patna and the Jesuits there to help her recruit anyone who might be willing to join the school. In July 1950, the school opened for its first official term with nine students from Calcutta, Bhuswal, Jamshedpur, the Santal Parganas, Bettiah, and Bangalore. They had come from all over India, a haphazard mix of whoever the sisters could find.

Lawrencetta was determined that the training at Nazareth Hospital would be equal in every way to that of nursing schools in the

United States. She set aside new rooms for the nurses on either side of the chapel on the upper floor of the convent building. The classes were carefully structured. The junior nurses took nursing arts, hygiene, anatomy and physiology, nutrition, bandaging, and drugs and solutions; the senior nurses took medical diseases, nursing care, materia medica, and operating room technique. Once a week, they all gathered for an ethics course taught by one of the Jesuits.

Lawrencetta decided she would have to design the nurses' uniforms herself. "The uniforms that the nurses have been wearing are not satisfactory," she wrote. "This new pattern should be more attractive and practical. Two caps were sent from the States so that we can make caps for the nurses like those worn by nurses in our training schools in America. Up until now the nurses have been wearing something that is like a probationer's cap." Within a couple of months, the darzi added the nurses' uniforms to his daily pile of sewing.

The frenetic pace at Nazareth Hospital that year comes through clearly in the Annals by September. Many of the entries discard the pleasantries and poetic descriptions of the plants and flowers during those brief few weeks of pleasant weather in the fall. "A very busy day." "These are very busy days in all departments." In one three-day period that month, the Annals noted that Florence Joseph and Ann Cornelius worked on an emergency surgery until 3:30 in the morning, and then continued into the following day for their next shift without any sleep. This was all while carpenters made tables and benches for the second-floor rooms, and electricians finished wiring the second floor, installing new lights on the roof and the stairway, and outlets in the rooms downstairs.

The electricity was run from a jury-rigged system: a diesel engine inside a cement and plaster powerhouse, from which they ran wiring to the house. The new government under Nehru was still a year away from the release of its first five-year plan, a bold attempt to turn India's wrecked agricultural economy into an industrial engine, and one of the first steps would be to add new power plants and extend their power lines beyond the big cities and factories. The electricity that ran those factories didn't come as far as the villages around Mokama. The sisters had been generating it all on their own—they added a second diesel motor to their powerhouse to run the electricity for the expanded hospital—but they could still run their fans for only a few hours a day. When the diesel engine broke down one summer, they had to send it to Calcutta for repairs and pray for cool weather.

There were rumors that this situation was about to change, with the construction of a new road and railway bridge across the Ganges, just a few miles from the convent. "There is a probability that we might get electricity, as this will be needed for the bridge building," the sisters wrote in a letter to the motherhouse. The sisters heard that engineers from America would soon arrive to lend their expertise, and they watched as tents for the project's foremen were put up on the railroad property adjoining the hospital compound.

The bridge promised a dramatic change to the character of Mokama. The Ganges had always been a hard border between the northern and southern parts of Bihar in that area, because there was no way to travel between them by train, truck, or car. Only the ancient river vessels could cross. To connect between the railway lines on either side, one had to leave the station on one side, wait for a ferry or barge to the other bank, and then board the train at a station on the other side. Dr. Lazaro and Babs made it a habit to drive the sisters to the ferry landing whenever they had to wait early in the morning. The journey from Mokama to Begusarai, a town just across the river, could take hours.

There was no running water to the convent either, and the sisters were reaching the limits of managing with the old-fashioned bucket well in the main courtyard. "A man is busy all day long carrying water from the well to the various parts where it is needed. He has a long bamboo pole which is put across the shoulders and on either end is attached a piece of metal to hold a bucket of water. He makes over a hundred trips a day, going back and forth carrying two large buckets of water each time." There were plans to bring water from a railway tank to a system of piped water for the hospital buildings. But the sisters would then have to bear all the costs of connecting the plumbing to bring it into the building.

It wasn't just electricity and running water. Like the rest of India, the people of Nazareth Hospital lived with constant shortages of the necessities of daily life. Indian factories were slowly building themselves up, but they were not moving fast enough to produce everything the new country needed or to meet the demand once filled by imported goods. Cloth and thread for uniforms and aprons were rationed and difficult to obtain. The sisters couldn't get jars for canning or jute for rope lines. The dhobis had to dry their clothes on the ground. Lawrencetta also gave up trying to procure certain scarce but necessary goods, like medical supplies, from America. The import duties were just too high. So she asked instead for money, figuring they would buy whatever was available locally, whenever they could.

There were chronic shortages of cement, coal, and iron. The sisters could stockpile steel, bricks, and rods, but they had to get a permit for cement and iron rods, a cause of chronic delays. And as she raced against the deadline for expansion, Lawrencetta realized that bricks, too, were not easily procured. "First of all, we have to make the bricks." They hired laborers to scoop up earth from the ground and form it into bricks by hand. "This takes a month or so and then two months to bake them and another for the kiln to cool off, so it is a good thing we have the extension of a year to fulfill the conditions."

The demands on the hospital, meanwhile, were never-ending. Another wave of refugees arrived in Mokama in 1950 after months of violence, mostly against Hindus, in what was then called East Pakistan. They were minorities in East Pakistan, and like Muslims and Anglo-Indians in India, had been under suspicion ever since Partition. By the end of 1950, hundreds of thousands of them had entered India as refugees. Most of these refugees went to West Bengal, but Mokama, too, had a refugee camp, which occupied the buildings of what had been the Ordnance Department. The doctor and a priest from Mokama visited and reported that there were about thirteen hundred men, women, and children in the camp and another five hundred at another camp nearby at Hathidah. Cholera had already broken out, and about twenty patients were isolated.

From the outside, the hospital looked like a chaotic mess. Scaffolding covered the front of the building, as two new floors were erected for the nurses' quarters, and patients sat waiting in any available space on the verandas and in the fields around the building. When the civil surgeon, inspector of hospitals for the region, paid a visit on September 4 to see the progress of the planned nursing school, he had some fairly obvious complaints to make: the hospital did not have enough beds, and only one doctor. He complained that "patients die because they are not attended to," a charge that the sisters found "absurd." As they put it in the Annals, "we would die ourselves before we would let them die for want of attention or care."

By December 1950, telephone poles were installed for first time in Mokama, one of them right in front of the hospital building. Phone service arrived soon afterward, and the hospital was assigned its own phone number: #3-Mokameh, Patna District. Lawrencetta was proud to describe the completed new structure for the nurses' quarters: a new wing of three floors that has "east and west exposure and gets a good breeze at all times."

On May 30, 1950, there was one instance when Dr. Lazaro went by himself to take the sisters to the ferry. The night before, less than six months after they had been married, Babs had suffered a miscarriage after a ten-week pregnancy. "We are all as grieved as she is," the sisters wrote in the Annals.

Soon afterward, the sisters learned that Dr. Lazaro had decided to leave Mokama to go to the United States. He had received a cable "confirming his appointment as a resident surgeon at St. Joseph's Infirmary in Louisville." Lawrencetta would not have been surprised; she encouraged his ambitions and likely helped him get the position at the hospital, which was closely associated with the order.

She wrote to her family in Louisville with the news, asking them to look out for him once he arrived in Kentucky. "He is a young man about 28, whose father is also a doctor. He is a very fine young Catholic, an ambitious and promising good surgeon, but doctors in this country do not have much of a name unless they have had some education in a foreign country." She told her family that she had given him their address and telephone number, and sent him with some snapshots of life in Mokama to share, and asked that they invite him to dinner and put him in touch with her brother who lived near St. Joseph's, so he would have somewhere to go on his time off. She tried to put them at ease. "He speaks English very fluently, but with a different accent than you are used to."

He was expected in Louisville on July 1, and Babs would have to stay behind in Mokama. Dr. Lazaro's last month in India was a flurry of activity. He and Babs went to Calcutta to complete his paperwork, and they made a trip by plane, a significant expense at the time, to see his relatives in Madras.

On June 20, the sisters hosted a farewell supper for him. He and Babs then took the express train for Calcutta, where he boarded a plane for London and then New York. Babs returned to Mokama a few days later and moved out of the hospital to stay with her family; Joe Gillard had, by then, been transferred to Mokama by the railways. Babs worked in the dispensary during the day and waited for word from her husband. The annals noted, "She is very, very lonely."

This was only the beginning of the farewells. Ann Roberta and Charles Miriam, who had been trained as teachers, had come to Mokama expecting that this new mission would, like every other mission opened by the order, include a school. That was their reason for being there. But vague plans to open a school in Bihar Sharif, a town connected to Mokama by rail, never materialized.

A letter from Ann Roberta records her disappointment: upon opening one of the many gift boxes of supplies sent to Mokama, she discovered, once again, that there was nothing intended for a school. "I claimed a little of everything and all the school materials for Bihar Sharif—or wherever we are to have a school. Alas and alack the others only laughed at me and now when nearly everything except the medicines, has been put to use or put away, there is no box with Bihar Sharif's name on it."

Of course, all the sisters kept busy. Ann Roberta spent a lot of time cooking. One Easter, she made "the first fried chicken that we have had in India," and four different kinds of candy, cake, and cookies. She became a special favorite of the orphans in the sisters' care and mastered Hindi, a skill that she was able to put to good use in the bazaar.

But it wasn't enough. In July 1950, Ann Roberta went over to the boys' school run by the Jesuits on the other side of the compound to teach two classes every morning and another after dinner. She taught reading, religion, Bible history, and drawing. The sisters had gone out of their way to maintain their independence from the Jesuits, insisting that they be treated as peers, with Lawrencetta and the order's leadership making all the decisions about the hospital. To allow one of her own sisters to work in that school, however close they might have been to the priests there, was a difficult compromise.

An unusual solution presented itself. In the fall of 1950, Lawrencetta returned from a trip to Patna with news from the bishop: the Loreto Sisters told the bishop that they no longer had enough people to continue running their school in Gaya and would have to give it up.

The school had been founded by a German order of nuns, the Sisters of Institute of the Blessed Virgin Mary, known in many places as the IBVMs. The order had been in Patna since 1853, having traveled across the country from Bombay by oxcart, and they started the school in Gaya, a few hours by train from Patna, in 1939. In 1943, the German sisters were detained in India as enemy aliens and turned over the running of the school to their Irish counterparts, the Loreto Sisters. By 1950, however, the Irish sisters were ready to give it up. After the war, young women seemed to have lost interest in following a vocation, and they did not have enough sisters to continue running the school.

The bishop accepted the Irish sisters' decision to leave, but he did not want to close the school altogether. It provided a crucial connection to the local elite of Bihar, who considered it a mark of status to send their children to a school run by Europeans. He asked the Sisters of Charity if they would take over.

It was an opportunity to do the teaching work they intended, without having to start from scratch, as they had with the hospital. The school at Gaya was already well established, with nearly 150 students—girls and boys, a population of mostly Hindus and a few Anglo-Indians—and a handful of lay teachers already employed. Lawrencetta went to Gaya and reported back that the sisters were asking an "extremely reasonable" price of 77,000 rupees for the property, a former Masonic lodge, and everything in it. All the sisters would have to bring with them were their toothbrushes. They waited for Mother Bertrand in Kentucky to make her decision.

A month later, it arrived. On November 16, a letter to Lawrencetta from the bishop reached the convent in Mokama. She happened to be in Patna that day, so the other sisters had to wait for her return to open it. But they had a clue: on the back of the envelope, as a postscript, were the words, "The school bus is yours too."

Ann Roberta and Charles Miriam immediately made plans to leave. The sisters made a short trip to Gaya to introduce themselves to the students and parents, and by the time they returned from the Christmas holidays in January, the Irish nuns had been replaced by two Americans. Ann Roberta took charge of the primary section, by far the largest department in the school, and Charles Miriam became the principal. They would be joined by two new sisters who were due to arrive from Kentucky at the end of the year. For all the joy and excitement of this new mission in India, the six pioneers also faced the reality that their original family had split apart.

Babs managed on her own in Mokama for about half a year, until the departure of the sisters to Gaya gave her a chance to find a new home. She taught the youngest children in the school in Gaya, with "forty little ones in her room." Dr. Lazaro found another position at Georgetown University and said he planned to return to India the following year, so even as she went about hiring a new interim doctor, Lawrencetta began putting aside cash and building material for a bungalow for the young couple. The constant shortages of cement delayed construction, but she continued little by little. "We hope to have the house ready when Dr. Lazaro returns," she wrote.

Eventually, he sent for Babs, who joined him in 1953. "Babs has at last gotten to America and is now happy with Doctor Lazaro in Washington. She had many disappointment [sic] and great anxiety in waiting." Once Babs and Dr. Lazaro were reunited in the United States, they made plans to visit the Veenemans in Louisville, but they postponed the trip when they discovered that Babs was pregnant again. Dr. Lazaro by then had been named chief resident at Georgetown, and their little girl arrived on January 19, 1954. "They have named it Erica. Both, mother and baby, were doing well when we heard. I know they are happy." Lawrencetta kept in touch with Babs and Eric Lazaro for years, long after it became clear that they would never return to Mokama.

TEN

The Frontier Women of Mokama

The difficulties of life in Mokama in the first years after independence—the lack of electricity and running water, the shortages of basic goods and medicines—were daunting but also exactly the sort of challenges for which the Sisters of Charity of Nazareth were well prepared. India demanded that they call on the original ideal of the order, that of the resourceful frontierswoman, to survive.

Of the six pioneers, Crescentia Wise was perhaps the one who embodied that model most completely. The entire hospital relied on her ingenuity to function. When Nazareth Hospital started doing surgeries, she figured out a way to provide running water so the visiting surgeons could scrub, as they were supposed to, under a continuous stream. "We can put a container of water upstairs in the dining room just over the OR, bore a hole through the floor, and run a rubber hose through it connecting the water and the basin in the operating room where the surgeon can wash her hands," Crescentia said. She added a sink to the medicine room, and another to the dispensary, and ran rubber tubing from it to drain the water outside. "Some day we will have running water but it is a big step forward to have a means of emptying water without running outside with it."

Crescentia suffered many illnesses—dysentery and dengue fever, as well as the alarming series of heart attacks—soon after she arrived in India, and yet during those early years she also found ingenious ways to collect rainwater and convert a pressure cooker into a still. She was certainly no stranger to hard work. Born Florence Rose Wise, Crescentia grew up on a farm in Stithton, in central Kentucky. She and her eight siblings enjoyed the simple comforts of that life—they had a proper house, owned cows and pigs, played baseball, went swimming in the nearby creek, and rode a mule to get around the property. The family's horse and wagon were reserved for early morning trips to Elizabethtown to shop.

But toward the end of World War I, in 1918, the United States Army acquired twenty thousand acres in and around Stithton to build what would eventually become Fort Knox. They paid off the Wise family and the other farmers, telling them they had the first right to buy back the land if the time ever came when the government didn't want it anymore. But that never happened. Her brothers and sisters scattered. Most of them stayed in Louisville, except for Maddie, who moved to Akron, Ohio, and Juanita, who went to Lebanon Junction. Soon after the army took over the land, Florence Rose entered the convent; and after the displacement of her family, she never looked back. She trained as a nurse and did just about every kind of nursing possible. She started with housework at Mercy Hospital in Mount Vernon, Ohio, even before she took her final vows, then moved to St. Joseph's in Lexington, where she did her training, worked in the operating room, trained other nurses, and then was put in charge of the "Colored Women's Ward."

She became a registered nurse in 1924, but wanted to do more, and the order needed pharmacists. She received her degree from the Louisville College of Pharmacy in 1937, the first of two women graduates from the college. A few months after graduating, she traveled to New York City for the annual meeting of the American Pharmaceutical Association, a gathering of enough significance to merit a story in *The New York Times*. The event was held at the Hotel Pennsylvania—the place made famous by Glenn Miller and Benny Goodman—and Crescentia was invited to present her paper on "parenteral" solutions, a new technology to get water and nutrients into patients. She argued that pharmacists shouldn't just leave it to big manufacturers to produce these solutions. They should be able to prepare them quickly and independently, whenever and wherever they are needed, because they are essential in emergencies.

Mokama put her theories to the test. The hospital needed distilled water, both for intravenous solutions and as a sterile solution to use during surgery. It was not possible to buy it, so Crescentia decided the sisters would have to make their own. She heated up water on a gasoline burner and then set up a still, like the ones she had seen around Nelson County, the birthplace of American whiskey. Her still was a tub of water on bamboo poles outside the dispensary window, with a length of rubber tubing, weighted down by a stone, through which the heated water slowly condensed and dripped back into the still. She collected rainwater from the roof and used it to distill enough sterile water to fill a hundred bottles for surgery and cleaning wounds. Until receiving a shipment of the standard "Baxter bottles" to dispense it for intravenous solutions, Crescentia used empty wine bottles instead; although the record does not specify where they came from, Communion wine from the Jesuits' supply is one possible source.

When the nursing school first opened for inspection, Crescentia took the opportunity of the civil surgeon's visit to secure an extremely precious commodity for the patients at the dispensary: morphine. Since the Opium Wars, it had been a highly controlled substance in India, so patients often suffered needless agony for the lack of legal painkillers. Crescentia filled out a stack of forms in advance to obtain a supply of morphine and other narcotics and asked him to sign it while he was there at the hospital. She was undeterred by his criticisms of the hospital; Crescentia simply ignored them. "He did not want to do it at all and tried in every way to refuse but Sister prevailed and the Civil Surgeon and those with him left in good humor," the Annals noted.

Crescentia's biggest triumph, however, was Nazareth Hospital's leprosy clinic. On the rough maps of the area around Mokama sketched out by Father Batson in his letters, he drew two small islands in the middle of the Ganges, little more than sandbars, labeled "leper colonies." There, people with Hansen's disease (named for the Norwegian doctor who in 1873 discovered the bacterium that causes it) lived apart from the rest of society. The practice of isolating patients with leprosy continued in India, even though by the late 1940s a new category of sulfa drugs had been shown to be extremely effective in treating the disease, particularly in its early stages, and were widely available in other countries. There were thousands of leprosy patients near Mokama with little access to treatment.

The presence of leprosy patients was actually a selling point for the order when Mother Ann Sebastian made the decision to send her sisters to India. "He even offers us a leper home in time, if you please, provided we are interested," Mother Sebastian wrote to the order, in her letter asking for volunteers. "The leper work is vast and most exciting, he says." For missionaries, working with leprosy patients was considered the most difficult work they could ever do, reserved for the elite few; it was a chance to use their medical skills, fill an unmet need, and in the process demonstrate the benevolence of God's presence.

The sisters procured hundreds of capsules of a sulfa drug called diasone and witnessed its effectiveness soon after the dispensary opened. An unsigned letter to the motherhouse in May 1949 described Roderick, a ten-year-old boy with leprosy who had been coming to the dispensary regularly to get his supply of the medicine. When he first came to the hospital, there were white patches on his face and a hard knot on his left cheek, his lips were thick and sore at the corners, and there were lesions around his nose. The diasone stopped the disease from getting any worse. "I am so happy about him because he already looks like a new boy," the letter noted. "His complexion this morning was flawless and everything about his face the reflection of a happy, healthy child."

By the end of 1949, the hospital's supply was running out; a donation of three thousand tablets languished for months while waiting for customs clearance in Bombay. A priest in Bhagalpur, a nearby mission, helped arrange a steady supply of diasone, but there were other obstacles to overcome: leprosy patients who came to the dispensary were shunned by everyone else because of the stigma around the disease. The stigma was so strong that the East India Railway allowed people with leprosy to travel for free to Mokama, without tickets. This meant that no one, not even a ticket taker, would be obliged to have contact with them. It would have been impossible, given her fragile health, for Crescentia to travel to all the remote villages around Mokama where leprosy patients lived in isolation. There was also no systematic way to make sure that those who came to the dispensary followed the prescribed two-week course of treatment.

Crescentia again found a solution: she decided to hold a regular free clinic at the hospital, taking advantage of its proximity to the railway station. She put out the word that Nazareth Hospital would hold the clinic on Wednesday afternoons, between the arrival of the morning train and the departure of the evening one, and she hoped the patients would come.

Crescentia's leprosy clinic began in the summer of 1952. She had a tabletop set up on portable bamboo poles, and she stood behind it with a box of medicines. There were tables and two chairs, one for the doctor and one for the nurse assigned to keep the records, and a shelter to give some shade from the midday sun. On the first day, there was only one patient. His name was Ram Dham, a man in the later stages of the disease. For weeks, he was the only patient. But he kept coming, and that alone gave Crescentia the courage to continue. As he improved, word spread quickly, and the crowds gathered every Wednesday.

She set up a system designed to handle hundreds of patients as efficiently as possible. On Saturdays, she enlisted the boys from the Jesuit school at Mokama and paid them a few rupees to put together packets: twelve diasone tablets, plus vitamins and iron pills, gathered in a small bag. After a few hours' work, the boys had prepared enough packets for the following week's clinic. Those who arrived on Wednesday were then divided into two groups. New patients went to see the doctor to evaluate them for symptoms of leprosy. Returning patients, who had already been diagnosed, would queue up in another line to see the two nurses. One would check their medical chart, the other would hand out a two-week supply of tablets.

As the crowds grew, Crescentia used wooden poles to mark off the queue, in a sometimes futile attempt to keep order. More important, she insisted on maintaining a clear record of who was being treated. Few of them had any kind of government identification, so she devised her own: a number issued to them by the hospital and kept on a card that they brought with them. That allowed Crescentia to keep track of who was coming regularly and who had missed a visit or tried to come before they were due. By November 1953, the clinic was treating 625 patients in a single day, with hundreds registered as regulars whose care and progress were being monitored. Soon afterward, the clinic grew to more than 1,000 patients a day.

Crescentia mobilized donations of medicine and cash to replenish her supplies of diasone, and in 1955 her work even enjoyed a brief moment of fame. The hospital at Mokama had no television, but according to the Annals, they received word from the motherhouse that Archbishop Fulton J. Sheen, the celebrity priest who had his own weekly show, *Life Is Worth Living*, had appeared on television and pledged that half the money he raised through the March of Dimes that year would go "to Patna for the lepers." It was a vindication of everything Crescentia had done in her long career and everything she believed the mission at Nazareth Hospital could do.

Crescentia represented the frontier resourcefulness that had animated the sisters' early history. But that was not the only model for how to be a missionary. The sisters were also bound by an ideal of modesty and piety that drew strength and purpose from the strict observance of the rule of hours and all the other regulations of being a sister. That model of missionary work was present in Mokama, too—in Lawrencetta's insistence on following the traditions of the motherhouse, in Florence Joseph's high standards in the hospital and nursing school, and in the quiet presence of Ann Cornelius Curran, the young sister who became the chief operating-room nurse.

Ann Cornelius was, in one respect, different from the other sisters at

Mokama. They had each been called to mission work for different rea-sons, but something in them wanted to extend themselves into the world—to be part of it, in a way that pleased God and fulfilled his will for them. But Ann Cornelius, even in India, seemed to look inward. She was meticulous and dedicated, and her work in the hospital was inti-mately connected to the work of contemplating what she had seen, the suffering and care and joy, and reflecting that back to God in prayer.

Born Martha Curran, she grew up in Bellaire, Ohio, a small town where her father ran a grocery store, the same one that his father had run before him. Her mother was a nurse from Columbus, Ohio, but she stopped working as a nurse once she started a family. The Cur-rans had ten children—including one who was stillborn, as Ann Cor-nelius learned much later, and her mother almost died during that birth. (Throughout her years in Mokama, the other sisters and nurses remarked on Ann Cornelius's soft spot for newborns. The annals noted that she was "very proud" of a premature baby who thrived in her special care and "went home a strong baby ready to begin life like anyone else.")

Among the many Curran siblings, Ann Cornelius was right in the middle. She had three older brothers, an older sister, and two sisters and two brothers younger than her. Their life in Bellaire was modest—they lived first in their grandparents' house, then in a rental on the edge of town. Their father drove them to school in the grocery deliv-ery truck and they walked home. Soon, they moved to another house, a smaller one, attached to the store. Their lives shrank to the five blocks between church, home, and school. Both her mother and fa-ther were passionate Catholics; they brought all the children to Mass every day before school, insisted that they come home every day for lunch, and said the Rosary with them every night before bed. Their father would bless them with holy water when he said good night, and their mother's great pride was inviting the parish priests over for dinner. "My Mother was a good cook and set a lovely table," one of the Curran sisters recalled years later.

Ann Cornelius was the quiet one of the four girls—she was the only one who said no to a date to the prom. (Even then, she knew that she wanted to be a nun.) And she was always the first to offer to help their mother. They were all close—there were only five years between the four girls—and they idolized the eldest, Ellen. She was an army nurse during World War II, and the other Curran girls wanted to be like her—daring, gregarious, and mature beyond her years. Ann Cornelius was the only one who came close. She and her sister, nicknamed Nancy, ended up joining the Sisters of Charity of Nazareth together, and Nancy adopted her adored sibling's name, becoming Sister Ellen. But Ann Cornelius is the one who became a nurse. She was a student nurse at St. Joseph's Infirmary during the war, and when the order declined the chance to go overseas, she took on the prestigious and difficult specialty of surgical nursing. And with her mission to India, she, too, managed to serve overseas.

By the time she left for Mokama, the family had moved to California, hoping to make a new start, so she had her farewell party there. Their father was so proud, and even Sister Ellen was granted some leave to wish her sister goodbye.

Ann Cornelius reserved a part of herself for her family. While she was known in the order for her prim demeanor, she had a sly humor that would occasionally emerge in the letters she wrote home to her sisters. She once wrote to her family that an area behind the hospital, planned for a vegetable patch, had been used as "an outhouse without the house so the soil should be good." And unlike many other nuns, she never used the name she took with her vows; she always signed her letters home "Martha."

At Nazareth Hospital, the operating room was Ann Cornelius's domain. She kept it in meticulous order, even before Nazareth had its own surgeon. She wasn't the one to be out in the courtyard with patients or haggling in the bazaar. She was close to Florence Joseph, who shared her insistence on high standards for the hospital, and took seriously the rule of hours as the only guide a sister in the order could need. Inevitably, the rule of hours came into conflict with the demands of running a hospital. This tension seemed to bother Ann Cornelius more than the other sisters; she wanted more time to pray, and she longed to be in a community oriented more clearly toward prayer and contemplation. For the first seven years of the mission, she endured that conflict and said little to anyone about it.

On January 1, 1954, the Annals recorded some baffling news: Sisters Lawrencetta and Ann Cornelius had gone to Calcutta to attend a religious exhibition, but only Lawrencetta returned. "When she left [Mokameh] the Sisters at the hospital didn't know she was leaving until they saw these men who carried the luggage to the railway, they came to the hospital and picked up a big box, a mattress and some other kinds of things. Those who saw it said, 'Whose is it?' 'What's happening?' So the buzz went around and then they found out that Ann Cornelius had left."

Only after she was gone did Lawrencetta make an announcement to the community: Ann Cornelius had traveled on from Calcutta to Dacca, in what was then East Pakistan, to enter the Franciscans of Perpetual Adoration Monastery, a cloistered order. She boarded a plane to Dacca on January 10. As adviser to all the sisters at Mokama, Lawrencetta must have planned the trip to Calcutta to make the sudden departure easier to bear for the other sisters.

When Ann Cornelius arrived in Dacca, the mother superior there welcomed her and told her that they thought it best for her to go into a retreat immediately. Ann Cornelius was to wear her own clothing during the ten-day retreat, and at the end she would be asked to wear the habit of this new community. The mother superior laid the habit across the chair in Ann Cornelius's room and left it there. On the last night of her retreat, as she was ready to turn out the light, Ann Cornelius looked at the Kentucky sunbonnet sitting there on the table, so stiff that it stood by itself, and said to herself, "I cannot leave it, I cannot leave it, I'll never leave it."

The next morning, she dressed as usual in her familiar habit and cap. When the mother superior came to the room to help her adjust the veil of the new habit, she was surprised to see this new recruit dressed just as she was when she arrived. Ann Cornelius told her she planned to return to Mokama, and the mattress and her trunk went back with her. When the train arrived at the station and the sisters heard the commotion of the porters carrying luggage, Florence Joseph sensed immediately what had happened. "That's got to be Ann Cornelius coming back, I knew she would return—I knew it!"

Ann Cornelius revealed later that the reason she could not stay in Dacca was more than just the habit. She went hoping for silence, a quiet space for prayer and contemplation; the observance of these new sisters included perpetual oral prayers, and she couldn't abide the constant sound. It would be another twenty years before Ann Cornelius would find the contemplative life she sought during that ill-fated trip.

The Annals of January 21, 1954, note that she has returned "home" to Mokama. "We are as happy as she."

ELEVEN

The Making of a Lady Doctor

I n the fall of 1953, another young doctor paid a visit to the Veene-man family in Louisville, and Lawrencetta's sisters immediately wrote back with the news. She had completed medical school at Georgetown in June and was about to start a surgical residency at the same hospital where the young priests on their way to India had stopped for their physicals. Louisville's *Courier-Journal* took note: "An energetic young woman at St. Joseph Infirmary is making religious history in the hospital's operating rooms." She wasn't just a doctor; she had also taken her vows as a member of the Sisters of Charity of Nazareth, and when her training was completed she would eventually be sent to Mokama. Here was the sister-surgeon that Nazareth Hospital had been waiting for.

Lawrencetta was thrilled to hear the news. "I am glad you got to see Dr. Wiss," she wrote. "Our new doctors are doing very well, but we wish she were with us. The time will pass quickly and she will be applying for her passport and visa before she realizes it."

The "new doctors" were the latest replacements for Dr. Lazaro, who had left Mokama for the United States in 1950. The hospital continued with a succession of substitute doctors, including some of Dr. Lazaro's classmates from medical school. There was Dr. Gernon, who "is doing very well but we think that he finds the people here a little undisciplined." Then Dr. De Silva, who began by visiting every other weekend while he finished training at Holy Family in Patna and eventually took over the post. "All three of these doctors are very good friends and all studied together at the Madras Medical College." Dr. De Silva later followed Lazaro's footsteps and left for a residency in Chicago.

Dr. De Silva was replaced by Dr. Smith, who served two years at Mokama and fit in well as a teacher and a physician but did not want to stay in Mokama. The sisters found a young Catholic couple, the D'Cunhas, both doctors, to replace him. "They are both very young," Lawrencetta wrote. They stayed for a while, and then came Dr. D'Cruze, another young Indian Catholic, who took over the doctor's bungalow with his wife and two young children.

The sisters, of course, had been looking for a female doctor, preferably a sister, since their first days in India. At first, Lawrencetta hoped she might find one among the doctors who were already in India, perhaps someone in Calcutta or Patna who might be tempted to come to a new hospital in a smaller town. But while she found some American dentists in Calcutta, including one who had done his training at Georgetown, they did not find any American physicians, nor could they find any Indian or Anglo-Indian lady doctors willing to join their new hospital.

It wasn't just the lack of trained women doctors in India; there were few doctors of any kind in India, and Nazareth Hospital struggled to keep competent doctors, who could easily find jobs in much bigger cities. Ann Cornelius, who rarely wrote to the motherhouse, explained in one such letter that the hospital in India was "completely different" from the ones where she had worked in Louisville. There, the order would send nurses to work alongside a staff of lay doctors, rather than just one or two. The sisters were able hospital administrators, and they were accustomed to hiring the doctors they needed as in-house staff—general physicians, as well as specialists in surgery and pediatrics, who could rotate shifts so one of them would always be on duty twenty-fours hours a day.

This was not possible in Mokama. There were a group of doctors in the town, but they had their own private practices in the bazaar and were not interested in becoming the employees of a group of American women, subject to night-time rotations and emergency calls. And without early training in a teaching hospital, they did not have the kind of wide-ranging expertise necessary to treat the people of Mokama. A staff doctor at Mokama might have to deliver a baby by caesarean section, diagnose a tuberculosis patient, and treat a farmer who had been headbutted by his buffalo all in the same day. "The few so-called doctors are not capable of handling every type of case, and nor can you depend on them for full-time duty," Ann Cornelius wrote. She concluded that "the biggest thing at the moment is the urgent necessity of having our own Sister doctors."

Sister Elise, a surgeon with the Medical Missionaries order at Holy Family Hospital in Patna, filled in whenever she could, and traveled to Mokama to handle complicated surgeries. As a stopgap, she gave the Kentucky nurses some essential surgical training. "She has let me do under her supervision everything she possibly could—things which are the work of doctors, but which she thinks I will be forced to do until we get a satisfactory doctor," Crescentia wrote in July 1948. "Yesterday she had me sew up (repair) a patient who was torn in delivery. Having done even this one will give me much more confidence."

That act skirted the boundaries of what was considered acceptable under canon law at the time, but the sisters realized it was necessary, and they could not have had better guides through that delicate territory.

The Medical Missionaries were the models for sister surgeons because they were among the first Catholic orders anywhere in the world to train their own sisters as doctors. To do that, they had to overcome centuries of patriarchal notions about what kind of work women in Catholic religious communities were allowed to perform. While professed sisters had been working within hospitals (and surely delivering babies) since at least the nineteenth century, the official Church position was that allowing religious women to be surgeons or midwives—professions that would put them in intimate contact with the body during childbirth—would somehow threaten their vows of chastity. This assertion of religious authority reinforced the gendered hierarchy of medicine, for it was doctors, and especially surgeons, who were considered the most powerful medical professionals in a hospital. The Catholic position on women in medicine was enshrined in canon law in 1917. The rule did not prohibit the practice of nursing, but it banned sisters from performing surgery or delivering babies.

The first challenge to this rule came from Dr. Agnes McLaren, the daughter of a prominent Scottish member of Parliament. One of the first women in Britain to qualify as a doctor, she was moved by the lack of medical care available to women in colonial India. In 1909, in the garrison town of Rawalpindi, she established St. Catherine's Hospital, intending to staff the hospital entirely with women doctors. She had heard of countless cases in which women suffered or died, especially in childbirth, because custom prevented them from being seen by a male doctor. The obvious solution was to hire women. But it proved to be almost impossible for her to find women physicians willing to serve in this remote outpost, so McLaren got trained help from a Franciscan missionary order. After working with them and discussing the problem with sympathetic priests, she became convinced that the only way forward would be to train a religious community of sisters as doctors who would commit themselves to work in mission hospitals. She would have to change canon law to make that possible.

McLaren, who had learned from her father how political pressure was built and deployed, enlisted support from the Church's missionaries. In the early twentieth century, missionary orders of priests were rapidly expanding into parts of Africa and Asia, and hospitals and schools were often the most effective and consistent way for them to meet potential converts. But as in India, in many of these places women would not see a male doctor. McLaren found allies among American, Irish, and Australian bishops, and together they lobbied the Vatican to obtain permission for professed sisters to become surgeons, midwives, and obstetricians as a way of advancing missionary work. McLaren, who was by then in her seventies, personally traveled to Rome five times to make her case.

In 1912, McLaren received an enthusiastic letter expressing interest in her work from a young Austrian woman named Anna Dengel, and she arranged for Dengel to begin studying medicine at University College Cork. McLaren died the following year, but Dengel completed her training as a doctor and carried on her mentor's work in Rawalpindi. She then traveled to the United States, which was becoming a center of power for the Church's missionaries, to build support among American priests who were sympathetic to the cause of allowing sisters to be trained as doctors. She got special permission to begin the Society of Catholic Medical Missionaries in 1925 with three other women, including one other doctor. Because they did not yet have the sanction of the Church, these women could not consider themselves full, "publicly" professed sisters—they had a separate status as missionaries. It took another ten years, but in 1936, with the publication of *Constans ac Sedula,* Pope Pius XI finally lifted the ban, and the Medical Missionary Sisters of Mary began their work in Rawalpindi and later in Patna, where they would serve as guides and advisers to the Sisters of Charity of Nazareth.

While the change in canon law was dramatic, different orders interpreted it differently. The Sisters of Charity of Nazareth took the narrow view that their order could not simply decide on their own to train a woman as a doctor; that work could only be done as part of sanctioned missionary work. Being a doctor, they believed, was not compatible with the other requirements of their ordinary rule of hours. As Dr. Wiss explained to the newspaper reporter: "It was church law until 1936 that sisters couldn't be doctors. It was felt that the two lives conflicted; a sister's life is so regulated and a doctor's life is so irregular." So when the order decided to accept the mission to India, although they had many highly qualified nurses and hospital administrators, because they had not yet accepted missionary work, they did not have any sisters who were trained as doctors. When Mother Ann Sebastian said yes to the Mokama Mission in 1946, she and her councillors began looking for someone who could begin training as a doctor right away.

They found her in Mary Wiss, a twenty-year-old novice from Columbus, Ohio, who played the violin beautifully and was about to begin working as a music teacher in Kentucky. When she entered the order in 1945, she had already finished most of her premed courses at Ohio State, but she felt called to be a nun and had left college to enter the convent. The Sisters of Charity of Nazareth was not a missionary order in 1945, so "it was a big decision for me, because I had always wanted to be a doctor, too."

After Mother Ann Sebastian made the decision to send the sisters to India, the leadership of the order came calling. (Lawrencetta, as leader of the Mokama mission would likely have known that Sister Mary Martha was in training, but there is no mention of her in the mission Annals for the first several years in Mokama.) The order asked for a significant commitment from Mary Martha. Would she be willing to finish her college coursework, begin medical school, and train to be a surgeon? It would take years of hard work, she would still have to follow all the rules of the order, and there were no guarantees. If things didn't work out for her in India, it would all be for nothing. She would be allowed to practice medicine only in the mission. If she came back, she could work as a hospital administrator, but her training as a doctor might go to waste.

Despite these warnings, Mary Martha was ready. "I was waiting for the chance to request permission anyway," she said. She made her first vows on July 19, 1947, and began her training at Georgetown University a month later.

Mary had been fascinated by medicine since she was a child, after her parents took in a boarder, a medical student, in their house near the Ohio State campus. Everything about it—the heavy books, the microscopes, the names of the strange diseases—captured her intense attention.

Her father, John Edgar Wiss, was born in St. Marys, a small town in northwest Ohio populated by German Catholic settlers, most of them farmers, who spoke German at home. (That stopped after World

War I.) John Wiss, whom everyone called Jack, went to Catholic
school and raced through everything the sisters gave him. He excelled
at German—they still taught it in school, and it was the language of
science and engineering at the time—and he started studying Latin
after the sisters noticed that he just didn't seem to have enough work
to keep himself busy.

Jack hoped to go to Ohio State, but his parents had no money for
the tuition, so after high school he started as a laborer at a factory
that made spokes for wagon wheels, the same one where his father
and brother worked. He handed over his salary to his mother to help
with the household expenses. But his mother had seen her son's intellectual promise, so she scrimped elsewhere and quietly saved all the
money he handed over. By the end of Jack's first year at the wagon
works, she had managed to save nearly all of it—about four hundred
dollars. She showed Jack's father the money and told him that was one
hundred dollars for every year, more than enough for tuition—it was
about fifteen dollars a semester for all the credits he could handle—
and his expenses. He could work for the rest if he had to.

Ohio was coming into its own as an industrial powerhouse, and
Jack Wiss could see that his future would not be made on a farm or
making wagons for farmers. He studied engineering, and while he
was there, he fell in love with a fellow student, Lucille Manney. She
was from a more prosperous family. Her father was a clerk at the
Ohio State Legislature and her mother was a telegraph operator, and
she had grown up in Cleveland. When the family moved to Columbus, Lucille cried at the thought of leaving cosmopolitan, lakeside
Cleveland for the "mudhole" that Ohio had chosen as its new capital.
They were close to Ohio State, though, and her father mortgaged his
house to pay for each of his children to attend, with the understanding that they would pay back whatever he had spent to educate them.

Lucille graduated with two degrees, in chemistry and science, and an engagement. Her parents were strict and frugal in their own way, and they would not allow her to marry until she had paid back her debt. She figured that if she taught at a convent boarding school all her expenses would be paid for, and she could pay her father back as quickly as possible. So Lucille headed to Kentucky to teach chemistry and home economics at the school run by the Sisters of Charity of Nazareth. Three years later, she returned, paid her debt, and married Jack in Columbus.

By that point, Jack was already working in Genoa, Ohio, as a chemical engineer for various gypsum companies. They sent him all over the Midwest, talking to clients and analyzing the raw material at limestone quarries that would eventually be turned into gypsum. He translated all the German works on mine chemistry into English for the company, and worked as a traveling salesman/consultant/engineer with a territory that at one point included five states—Ohio, Indiana, Pennsylvania, Michigan, and parts of Kentucky.

After the Great Depression, most of Jack's unit was laid off, but they kept him on. He was willing to do the work of several people—engineer, stenographer, salesman, and materials chemist—and he never seemed to slow down. After a major heart attack, he needed a hobby to keep his hands and attention occupied. He started planting flowers, and soon spent much of his free time weeding the flower beds, tending roses, and nurturing the delicate orchids that became his pride and joy.

The family lived in Chicago briefly, during the heyday of "mob rule" in the 1920s. Lucille gave birth to a son, John Jr., in 1924, but was attended by a careless doctor and nearly died in childbirth. When she became pregnant again, she went to her parents' house for her confinement. The doctor told her she hadn't been stitched up properly after her first delivery, so in addition to delivering a baby girl, Mary, he also repaired some of the damage that the first doctor had done.

Mary was a difficult baby. She had colic, and cried and cried and cried. For months it went on. The neighbors could hear her wailing in the night. They told her mother that she would never raise that child. They meant that the child wouldn't survive. They took colic to be a sign of sickliness and ill luck. But her mother was determined to prove them wrong. She did, and had another daughter, Martha, soon afterward.

While her husband traveled, Lucille managed the house and three young children by herself, despite chronic poor health. She was often so weak that she would need two hands to hold up a cup of tea. Eventually a doctor figured out what was wrong when she brought the two older children in with what turned out to be misdiagnosed scarlet fever. The doctor noticed that Lucille was severely anemic and had been for years. He gave her an "iron tonic," and she later had an operation for cancer. She was told she could not bear any more children.

Lucille hated the big city—she did not want to raise her children in a place where they picked up low-class habits like sitting outside on the curb—so she sent them every summer either to St. Marys, where the Wiss family farm still used a horse-drawn plow, or to Columbus, to visit her parents. Lucille was thrilled when U.S. Gypsum transferred them to Columbus. But then, surprisingly, she got pregnant again when her three other children were all teenagers. The doctor ordered bed rest for the entire pregnancy, and her oldest daughter, Mary, took over the running of the household, doing the cooking and cleaning in addition to attending high school.

Mary Wiss had grown into her father's daughter. She was tall and tough; if anybody bothered her siblings, she was the one to handle the bullies. She knew her own mind and didn't like to be told what to do.

People told her she could be overbearing, but she didn't care. It was just a matter of getting the job done. At nearly six feet tall, she felt matronly in the clothes that fit her in ladies' boutiques, so she made her own. She liked the crowd in her brother's high school class better, so she skipped a grade and graduated with them.

She knew she wanted to be a surgeon, a doctor who would care for women like her mother in the way that they deserved. But the nuns were the ones who pushed her and encouraged her in school, and she wanted to be part of their community. Maybe she could be a doctor and a nun. Never mind that women in that era did not do both.

When Mary finished high school in 1942, at sixteen, she told her mother she wanted to join the convent. She was too young, her mother said, so Mary enrolled at Ohio State, in premed. But her calling eventually became too strong to ignore. With World War II still raging in Europe, she left for Kentucky to join the Sisters of Charity.

She knew the order well. Her mother had worked at the academy in Nazareth as a teacher, and the sisters had run the grade school in Columbus. But she needed a letter of recommendation from the parish priest. Monsignor Nolan was a sour, ill-tempered man. He was familiar with the order—they had taught in his parish school—and there was something about them that he didn't like. "Why would you want to do that?" he asked her. He refused to write Mary a letter.

She would not be deterred. She called up the mother general and said she really did want to come but could not get a letter from her pastor, Monsignor Nolan. Oh, we know him, they told her, don't worry about it. Mary Wiss entered the convent on January 18, 1945, and received her habit soon after.

On a visit home, she found that her parents, too, had taken on a mission of a sort. The Midwest was full of refugees from World War II, and Catholic Relief Services was looking for people to house them.

With two children graduated and out of the house and plenty of room at home, Lucille and Jack Wiss took in two young men who had been soldiers in the Mikhailovich army and had just enrolled at Ohio State. Mary greeted them and went out to the backyard to help pull weeds with her father.

Although the order had gotten special permission to send Mary to medical school in Georgetown, the rules of the order still applied. She had to devote time to prayer and daily Mass as she always did. And she had to wear the habit all through medical school in spite of how uncomfortable it was; she used to joke that you could hide your lunch under there. The stipend she was given was never enough—she had to borrow sometimes to get through the day—but she enjoyed medical school and got along with her classmates. She laughed at their pranks and practical jokes, like the time she discovered a giant cockroach in a six-inch-long test tube. Someone had put it there and labeled it "Delivered in ward x"—the maternity ward—to watch her reaction.

They called her "Super Stitch." All those years sewing her own clothes had turned her into an able seamstress, and the fine work of a surgeon came easily to her. On the day that she took the Hippocratic oath, she stood in the back, tall and serious, her black habit and white Kentucky sunbonnet only slightly out of place among the dark academic robes the rest of the students put on for the ceremony.

She was the first female surgeon in Kentucky certified by the American Board of Surgery, and in July 1953 became a resident at St. Joseph's Hospital in Louisville. During her years of training as a surgeon—while the hospital, the nursing school, and the leprosy clinic in Mokama were coming into their own—Dr. Wiss found a comfortable place among the other surgeons. She had colleagues whom she would remain close to for decades, and she was able to devote herself completely to developing the skills she would need in India. They made sure to train her for everything she could possibly need to know, like how to read X-rays, although that wasn't something surgeons usually did. She would be the chief surgeon at Nazareth Hospital, of course, but everyone at St. Joseph's also knew that she was heading to a mission serving tens of thousands of people, where she would often be the only doctor available.

TWELVE

Women of the New India

M any of the first nursing students in Mokama came from a small community of Anglo-Indians. The Annals of January 1951 recorded some of their distinctive names, which reflect their European and Indian heritage: Sheila Michael, Joan Blacquiere, Florence de Cruz, Barbara Alasia, Lily Andrews, and Iris Hardinge. It was not surprising that the sisters found their first students in this community. Nursing was a well-regarded profession among them, and the figure of the Anglo-Indian nurse appeared regularly in the popular culture of the time—glamorous, high-spirited, and free from the conservative norms of Hindu or Muslim society.

But after Partition, Anglo-Indians began to leave India, and Anglo-Indian nurses disappeared from India's hospitals. As word began to spread about the nursing school in Mokama, South Indian women took their places. By July 1954, when a new class of fourteen entered the nursing school at Mokama, nearly all of them were South Indian, mostly from the state of Kerala. They had learned about the hospital through word of mouth, whether from parish priests or at gatherings of the Catholic Hospital Association or the Trained Nurses Association of India, in which the order had started to become active.

Two kinds of young women from Kerala answered the call. The first were those who chafed at the restrictions of their conservative society. Unlike Anglo-Indians, this Christian community was insular and observed many of the same traditions—including arranged marriages, dowry, and caste prejudices—as their Hindu neighbors. They were privileged and had a comfortable position, but they wanted something more. And then there were those who knew they would never fit into the rigid structures of the society—fatherless and motherless children, who would have to find their own place to belong. A generation earlier, the best they could hope for was a fortunate marriage, a kind man who would take pity on them and marry despite their poor prospects. But now this American nursing school was offering something else—a way out.

Kerala was home to an old and storied community of Indian Catholics, and therefore a natural choice as a place to recruit nurses. Three of the sisters had already been there, on their initial voyage to India, when the *Steel Vendor* made port at Cochin. They got off the ship and spent a few days in this historic town, a jewel on the spice route and a destination for explorers from Vasco da Gama to Ibn Battuta. They saw convents, hospitals, and schools run not by American nuns but by Indian Catholics, a small and well-established minority who proudly, if apocryphally, traced their heritage back to the wanderings of St. Thomas the apostle, who supposedly converted a group of Brahmins.

There is no clear evidence of such an encounter, but there is a record of Christians from the Middle East arriving in 345 AD to escape persecution by the Sassanid Empire (like the Catholics who settled in

Kentucky, who had fled persecution in England). Aramaic or Syriac was their language of worship, and ever since then the community has been known as Syrian Christians. There were splits among them over the course of many centuries, as some aligned themselves with the Eastern Orthodox Church and some with Protestants, but Syro-Malabar Catholics, who stayed loyal to Rome, became the largest group of Syrian Christians, about 40 percent of the Christian population in the region and a powerful political and economic force.

In November 1954, having trained a handful of these young women from the south, the sisters decided to make their case directly to them. Crescentia and Florence Joseph went to Bangalore for a meeting of the Catholic Hospital Association, and then Bombay, to attend the National Marian Congress, and they returned to Mokama on December 10. During this time, they also likely made their first recruiting trip to the south. (An account of their trip there is recorded in one of the order's mission histories, although no date is given.)

They were impressed by the Catholic schools, hospitals, and colleges, which were nothing like the ones in Bihar. They were full of educated young women and pastors who welcomed them and promised to promote their work. They arranged for Crescentia and Florence Joseph to visit convent schools to make their pitch for the Nazareth School of Nursing in Mokama. "They explained to the girls that, in gaining nursing skills, they could not only help the needy of the North but also acquire for themselves a professional skill leading to social independence," according to an account of the trip. That message landed with unusual power. The world of the Syro-Malabar Catholics was changing in every possible way—pulled apart by the same forces changing India. And the women the sisters encountered in Kerala were changing with it.

One of them was Bridget Kappalumakal, who was born in 1937 on one of the lush, tropical estates that covered the central part of Kerala, in a village called Meenachil, named after the river nearby. It was about two miles from the church and shops in the nearest town, Palai, in the heartland of the Catholic community in Kerala.

Bridget's family was counted among the landed gentry, who had gained a particular power and status through the institutions of Church schools and colleges. Her father owned about sixty acres of land, made wealthy by rubber, coconut, areca nut, black pepper, coffee, tea, and turmeric. They grew more than enough for the family to eat, and rarely had to buy anything from outside, a mark of wealth and comfort in Kerala. There were always at least two or three laborers living in a small shelter on the land and two women who helped with the housework, although they returned to their homes in the evening.

Although her family was not Brahmin, they owned land and did little to challenge the brutal hierarchies of caste. In many Syrian Christian families, if an outcaste, a pariah, approached the house and asked for water, a servant would take a steel cup kept aside for that purpose and pour water from the well into this cup and offer it to them. The touch of a pariah on a family's well would leave it, in their eyes, irredeemably polluted.

Bridget was the seventh of eleven children, all but two of them daughters. Her eldest sister married when Bridget was still a toddler, and had children soon afterward, so her playmates included nieces and nephews not much younger than she was, all living on a big family compound, full of children. They spent most of their time running around the property, making up games. They ate their meals outside;

she could roam for hours and rarely see anyone outside her own family.

They lived in a big teak house, with six bedrooms, a dining room, and a kitchen. There were coconut trees everywhere—so many that the family could eat their fill, use the shells for fuel and the husks to make coir, and still have hundreds left over to store in the attic. Once a year, her father would arrange to sell the entire inventory. They kept a stash of sprouted coconuts in the attic, too. Those were stored until they began to flower and the coconut water was absorbed by the plant, turning the whole fruit into coconut "pong"—a spongy treat, something like a cake, with a more delicate taste.

Bridget's father, the oldest of all his brothers, had done well for himself. He studied only until the seventh grade and then left to help take care of his father's estates. When it was time for him to be settled, he took the property he inherited, including the house built by his grandfather, and expanded it. Bridget admired him. She was the one, of all her sisters, most likely to be his shadow, to go with him as he methodically walked through the property, checking on the progress of the rubber plants, directing the laborers while she watched and listened, chewing on pieces of tender coconut.

He had one wish, that all his children would be better educated than he was. So he sent them to the Catholic schools nearby. They walked to school and back, and studied at home by the light of a kerosene lamp in the evenings, then said prayers for an hour before bed. There were rare breaks in the routine; during school vacations or on feast days, her sisters' children would come to visit or they would go to her mother's family home.

Not even independence interrupted their idyll, or the political struggle that followed, or the labor agitations and strikes of the 1950s, as the Communists offered an outlet for people's frustrations with the

Congress Party. Bridget and her family were insulated from it all on their estate, set back from the river and protected by the coconut palms. By the time Bridget finished high school, people were out in the streets, shouting slogans against the government, and some of her friends were put in jail. Her father got the Malayalam newspaper and read it every day, but he never talked to Bridget about what was going on. She had never been farther than ten miles from her own house, at the edge of her grandparents' property, but she knew that something was happening, something in the world beyond her.

Bridget was impatient. Her older sister was finishing high school and was about to join a convent in Delhi. Everybody knew she would be a nun from the very beginning. She was so pious, so holy. Bridget was different, "a more worldly girl." She was proud of her thick, glossy hair, which reached below the curve of her waist. She liked to go out, in mixed groups of boys and girls, especially to the movie house in Palai. She was very particular about her food; simple vegetarian rice and curry wouldn't do. She wanted fish or meat at every meal and liked to have it served on time. Her sister, on the other hand, seemed indifferent to pleasure of any kind. She didn't care, and would eat anything without complaint.

When Bridget finished school, she told her parents she wanted to become a nun. She asked her sister if she could go with her to the same convent, but her sister refused. She didn't think Bridget would survive the homesickness and isolation and suspected she would give up at the first difficulty. If Bridget gives up and leaves the convent, she said, "it will reflect badly on me." She told Bridget to try another convent—one in the south, closer to home, something easier—and said to their father, "She's not meant to be a sister."

Bridget didn't care. She knew only that she wanted something other than the path laid out for her, married life in Meenachil or a village just like it nearby. High school went through class eleven, then there were two years of college, and at the end of that, either you got married or you became a nun. She had already seen everything there was to see about life in Meenachil: cooking and children and church, nothing else. If she stayed, she would end up living on her parents' property, just as they lived at the end of their parents'.

She went to the priest who had helped to arrange her sister's assignment and told him that she, too, had a vocation, but she wanted to go to Patna. She had read about the work of the Patna Mission in the magazines published by the Jesuit missionaries and imagined herself doing heroic work among the "pagans" of North India. It was the hardest work you could do as a nun, and Bridget was determined to conquer it. The priest took down her name and told her he would let her know. She waited. She passed her exams, and still she didn't hear anything.

Eventually, Bridget received word from the priest. He had found her a place in Mokama. He told her the convent was near Patna and that it was started by American nuns who were running a nursing school, so she would get some training and eventually join their order. But she would have to decide quickly. He was organizing a group of girls to meet at the train station in Ernakulam, a big city on the coast, and they would leave in five days' time.

Bridget's father didn't want to let her go so far from home. He said Bihar was too poor and too backward, nothing like Kerala. He wanted her to go to college. She was well educated, from a wealthy family. And her older sister, the one who everyone knew was meant to be a nun, was already joining a convent. Why would she want to waste her life in some desolate part of North India?

She was determined to persuade them in the few days she had before the train would leave. Her mother agreed, but her father was unyielding. Bridget announced a hunger strike and finally her father relented. (Her brother predicted that she wouldn't last long in Bihar anyway.) Bridget knew what she was getting into. The priest had explained to her that when you went on a mission, you would never see your people again. Bridget was ready.

The train made its way east across the Nilgiris, the blue hills that separated Kerala from Tamil Nadu. From there, it headed down toward the coast, to Madras. They had to change trains there, and while they waited the priest took them down to the beach to see the ocean for the first time. The hugeness of it—the waves gathering force, racing toward them like rockets, crashing against the sand and then pulling out and heading toward them again—the drama and power of it stunned her. Some of the girls were scared. But Bridget joined hands with three of the others and marched toward the sea. They turned their faces to the waves and walked into the water until the hems of their saris were soaked.

Bridget, who arrived in Mokama in July 1955, was among the first group of young women to respond to the sisters' call for recruits. There were many more that followed. In the years afterward, labor agitations began to stifle daily life in Kerala. The Syrian Christians could see what was happening; their position of privilege in Kerala was at risk. The Communists were opposed to religion and the Church and hostile to landowners, the organizing principles of their lives. They were the ones with the most to lose if the Communists came to power.

Many thousands of Syrian Christian men began to leave Kerala during this period, seeking opportunity in the big cities of India and in some cases abroad. Perhaps more surprisingly, young women did, too. The Diocese of Palai, where Bridget grew up, was the center of Catholic life in Kerala, and the parish priests became their allies. The recommendation of these powerful men helped persuade the conservative families who were reluctant to send their daughters so far away. Some of those daughters did not necessarily have a call to become nuns but were instead drawn by the chance to become nurses—a profession that, at least in their community, had begun to shed some of its stigma.

Rose was one of these girls. She grew up in a village not far from Bridget's. She was named after her mother, but everyone called her by her nickname. She was the baby, a little girl doted on by everyone around her from the minute she was born, just before Easter in 1943.

Independence was an early, dim memory for Rose. She remembered seeing the adults gripping the precious ration slips for cloth and rice and sugar—and then one day all that tension was released in a burst of fireworks and commotion and cheering crowds on the road.

Like Bridget's, Rose's childhood world did not reach past the boundaries of her family's estate. Her older siblings, three sisters and three brothers, were always there to play with her among the coconut trees, especially the twin brothers just two years older than her. Almost everything they needed, her family grew or raised on the acres of rainforest around their house: rice, jackfruit, mangoes, coconut, vegetables, pepper, spices, coffee, chickens, cows, a pig, a goat. The only things they bought from the market were fish, tea, and sugar.

Rose was strong and as soon as she could walk she would run to keep up with her brothers. They walked the two miles to school together six days a week, splitting up once they reached the main road, because her brothers went to the boys' school and she went to the convent school for girls. They came home for lunch and then went to church for catechism. It was almost dark, around 5:30, when they returned home.

She learned early that there were certain tasks reserved for girls. They all had chores, but the ones for girls were meant to train them for marriage. Otherwise, she was told, when you get married and go to another house, you will not know what to do. So she swept the front yard, picked mangoes and dried the mango pulp in the sun to make thera, a mixture of dried mango and coconut reserved for company. In the evenings, there were animals to tend.

They didn't have a radio or television, so their main entertainment was church on Sundays. They would go to catechism afterward and have a glorious hour or two to see their friends. After church, the family would walk home. There wasn't time to do much after that, other than wash and iron the school uniforms to prepare for Monday.

The biggest adventure for Rose and the twins was summer vacation, when one of them—they had to take turns—would make the trip to see Achayan. He was their oldest uncle, and he lived with his wife in an even more remote village, managing a pepper estate. When it was Rose's turn to visit, she would start in the morning, walking three or four miles to catch a bus, riding the bus until the road ended, and then walking to the river Pampa, close to Achayan's house. There was no bridge, so she would wait for the boatman to take her across, before walking the rest of the way to get to the house by evening. She spent the days there picking ripe papayas off the trees, looking for snakes in the tall grass, and swimming in the river.

Every month, Achayan would come to Rose's house for a few days. Those visits were different. There was some unspoken anger. Achayan always needed money; it took years to grow pepper plants, and many men to cultivate them, so he would come to ask for money to pay the workers and buy rice and all the other provisions they couldn't get on the estate. His wife rarely came; she went to another house nearby.

By the time she was about ten, Rose somehow figured it out. Achayan and his wife weren't her uncle and aunt. They were her parents. Her grandparents had been raising her, and the siblings she was so close to were in fact her uncles and aunts.

Eventually, she learned the story. Her father was the oldest of seven, so he was the first to be married, and Rose was born a year later. His family followed the traditions of the landed gentry of Kerala: before the second son was married, they would settle the oldest on his own property, so he could have his own household, and the family could avoid the inevitable conflict among daughters-in-law.

In some families, the oldest sons moved into a house near the parents. But Rose's father was an alcoholic, and his parents wanted to keep him as far away as possible from the rest of the family. They didn't want to make it more difficult for his three sisters to be married off, so they found him an estate many miles away. Before Rose was two years old, her parents left. In her grandparents' home, at least, she would have other children to play with, and her mother would have to manage only a volatile husband on that remote patch of pepper. Rose became the baby of the house, assuming that her uncles and aunts were her siblings. Eventually, her parents had another daughter, and another. One by one, the new children came to live with her in the family compound.

By the time she was eighteen, she had four younger sisters and realized it was up to her to take care of them. Her father's alcoholism had gotten worse. No one could control him, and it was bad enough that he could no longer manage the estate. He moved back to his parents' village and lived in a small house nearby. But he took no responsibility for his daughters, and Rose continued to live with her grandparents.

She thought to herself, I have to make my own living. I can't depend on my father. I will have to leave.

When Rose was a girl, everything outside their village—and certainly outside the world of Malayalam-speaking Catholics—was foreign to her. In her mind, she tallied up everyone she knew who had left. She had an aunt—one of the girls she thought of as her sister—who had become a teacher and a couple of classmates who had started teacher training. But Rose had no money for the fees. She had an uncle who became a college professor and another who went into business. But she was terrible at math—Rose was worried she might not even finish high school—so she ruled that out. Her other two sister-aunts had married into landed families. Rose, too, could have stayed in Kerala and married, but how would she support her sisters? She had seen a few girls who became nuns, but there was obviously no money in that.

She had heard of young women, a few years older than herself, who had gone to Kuwait and Persia to work as nurses. They came back for their annual vacations wearing colorful saris, their long hair teased into glamorous, complicated styles, and would leave behind perfume and presents for their families. Rose had no idea what nurses actually did. She had seen one or two at the local hospital, on a Sunday visit to a sick relative, and the ones who helped her when she was admitted once with a stubborn fever. But they were really just assistants, the girls who might have done a local six-month course. Rose wanted more.

She knew of one other girl from her village, older by a few years, who had gone to study nursing in a proper course somewhere in North India. And she heard that some of these nursing programs didn't require fees, so she wouldn't have to ask her father or anyone else for money to pay for it. In fact, she thought she would get a stipend, as they did at government hospitals. Surely this was her path out of Palai. As soon as she got her high school certificate (she barely passed), Rose found out the name of the priest who had helped another girl leave and went to see him. He lived in Bharananganam, a village about five or six miles away by bus. She needed a chaperone, so she convinced one of her uncle-brothers, who always indulged her, to go with her.

There were one or two other girls waiting outside Father Sebastian Pinakat's office when she arrived. Rose hadn't made an appointment, so she waited. He was in his sixties, a longtime parish priest with many contacts among the Jesuit missions in Patna and Mokama. For years, he had been encouraging young women with a vocation, or even just curiosity about the world outside Kerala, to try Mokama.

Father Pinakat explained to her that there were government hospitals, there were mission hospitals like the one she had seen, and there was Mokama. He looked at her high school certificate, told her she could apply to a few different places, gave her the forms, and explained how to complete them. She would need a medical exam, a chest X-ray, blood tests, and certificates showing that she was a Catholic and that she had passed high school. He didn't really ask any questions; the whole thing was over in forty-five minutes.

Her uncle did all the paperwork; she had no idea how to write a letter or how to address one. She never had any reason even to write a letter—her whole world was there at home. Within three weeks, she got a letter accepting her to Mokama. She told her grandparents she just needed to get out, and her uncle lobbied for her. They were comforted by the fact that there was at least one other person from their village there, and that Father Pinakat had given his blessing.

Her grandfather didn't say much, but he agreed without protest to pay for all the things she would need in her metal trunk. The nuns had given them a detailed list—five white saris and matching blouses, several sets of underwear and stockings, a thin mattress and sheets, a comb, brush, toothpaste, and other personal things. She got word from the priests that there were two other girls from Palai who were also going, and she was to meet them in Pravithanam, a village close to theirs, and travel together. Classes would begin on August 1.

On July 26, two months after graduating from high school, Rose prepared to leave. Someone had warned her she might not like the food, so she carefully packed some pickles made from the limes and mangoes grown on her family's estate in her trunk next to the saris. She still wasn't used to wearing them. Girls in Kerala wore long skirts and cotton blouses; the last time she had worn a sari was at her graduation ceremony, so it still felt like playing dress-up. But she knew she had to get used to it, so she wore a new colored sari for the trip.

At the station, her uncle gave her the usual advice—listen to the nuns, work hard, behave well, don't bring shame to the family. Rose noticed that most of the other girls were crying, embracing their parents until the last possible moment. Rose didn't feel like crying. She was sad, but more than that, she was struck by a feeling of just not knowing what was going to happen. And she couldn't stop staring at the train; it was the first time Rose had ever seen one.

They had plenty of chaperones along the way. One girl's father went with them as far as Madras, where he happened to meet some Indian nuns, who went with them as far as Calcutta. The sisters had some extra rosaries in their bags, and before they left the station, they insisted that the girls wear them, to give the impression that they were also nuns and perhaps avoid the attentions of young men on the train. It was their second night traveling, and Rose was too tired to argue. The sisters put them on the night train to Mokama, and they arrived at about four in the morning, tired and dirty.

Two older students met them at the Mokama railway station. One of them scoffed at the rosaries as soon as she saw the new girls climbing off the train. Take those off, she told them. And they followed her the rest of the way.

What, then is the use of allowing a woman to go outside the home? . . . A daughter must be settled early in life. If we allow her to roam about too long, she will perhaps become discontented with her fate, and the sin of it will be on us.

RUTH PRAWER JHABVALA, *THE NATURE OF PASSION*

THIRTEEN

The Novices Go on Strike

B y 1955, the women of Nazareth Hospital were a completely different group from the "six pioneers" who had arrived together on those two ships. Charles Miriam and Ann Roberta had left Mokama and were teaching in Gaya. The order had sent new batches of missionaries from Kentucky to help with the school in Gaya and the hospital in Mokama, and some of them traveled by airplane rather than by ship. Lawrencetta was still in charge, but the configuration of their work had changed. Florence Joseph had more help on the nursing wards, so she spent much of her time managing the new sisters and the nurses in training. Ann Cornelius was often called away to help teach in Gaya, and Crescentia was busy running the leprosy clinic.

Mokama, too, had changed, as Nehru's grand plans for industrialization slowly took shape. The hospital received its first phone call—"the operator ringing to see if his call came through all right"—and rural electricity finally reached Mokama, so the sisters got rid of the diesel engines that had powered their lights and fans for nearly a decade. They had piped running water in the hospital and even in the bathrooms, a welcome improvement after the intermittent cholera epidemics in Mokama, which sickened some of the sisters along with everyone else. Nehru had to raise tax money to pay for all this progress, as the sisters learned when Mokama was designated as a "Notified Area." The hospital would be expected to pay tax, although they tried to get an exemption.

The shortages of manufactured goods, including medical supplies and equipment, persisted, but the sisters found new ways to get what they needed. The United States had been able to negotiate a humanitarian exception to the high duties imposed on foreign goods, so shipments sent to Mokama through the National Catholic Welfare Conference would be exempt from import duties. The U.S. government and the newly formed organizations of the United Nations were also making more of an effort to help India. Sister Crescentia came back from a meeting in Calcutta with a movie projector donated by the United States Information Service; in 1955, UNICEF and the National Catholic Welfare Council came to visit Mokama firsthand to see what the hospital needed.

None of these changes were as profound or as difficult, however, as the arrival of Indian women hoping to become nurses and professed sisters at Nazareth. Their presence would challenge every assumption the American women had about why they had come from Kentucky and what their place in India was meant to be.

Bridget's group of five was among the first to arrive. In her zeal to leave home, she did not really know what she would be doing once she got to Mokama or who would be in charge. She imagined that when she arrived at the station, she would be greeted formally by women in black habits, her guides to the strange world of "pagan" North India. But when she reached the station, there was no one but a servant sent to meet her and the other girls and lead them on the old path through the railway colony to the convent. Her disappointment turned to despair. "We got to the convent, they turned around, and we saw them. They were all wearing white. And they were white."

Until that moment, it had not truly sunk in that she was joining an American congregation or that she had left her family to live with a group of white American women. They began speaking to her, but none of the words directed at her seemed to have any meaning. She couldn't even tell if they were Hindi or English. The sounds were so completely different from the Malayalam she knew as her first language, and they didn't seem to match the textbook Hindi and English she had studied in school. Bridget tried to follow along, replying "Yes, sister," and "No, sister," to whatever she heard. And she followed obediently when they sent the five young women to the nurses' quarters.

Lawrencetta, too, was not quite sure what to do with Bridget and the rest in that first group of candidates, who wanted to enter the order as novices. She had been corresponding with her superiors at the motherhouse for years about the possibility, and in October 1954, she wrote, "Yes, we will start a novitiate here as soon as we get permission from Rome. There are many vocations in the south, where the Catholics date back to the time of St. Thomas." But Lawrencetta received no guidance, and she was not sure how Indian women would fit into their order and the work they were doing.

There were few precedents to guide her. There was the order established by Mother Teresa, who began her work in Calcutta at about the same time that the Kentucky sisters arrived. They kept in close touch, and in April 1951, Sister Crescentia traveled to Calcutta "for the clothing ceremony of Mother Teresa's first postulants." But that was a new community established in India, not an American order with its own history and traditions. The Sisters of Charity had come to India to serve the poor with hospitals and schools—not to find new sisters of their own.

There were some South Indian orders in Kerala among the old Indian Catholic communities; one of them, the Sisters of the Adoration of the Blessed Sacrament, sent two of its members for nursing training in Mokama in August 1952. And then there were the various "native orders" of Catholic sisters, communities of exclusively Indian nuns who were affiliated with European missionary orders. The sisters from Nazareth encountered them often, but Lawrencetta found the arrangement disconcerting. When the Sisters of Notre Dame, whom she knew from the annual retreats in Darjeeling, began a novitiate for Indian women, Lawrencetta went to a ceremony marking the occasion of the first postulates receiving their habits. She noted that the new novices "looked like little dolls dressed up" because they were so much smaller than American women.

Without explicit permission from the motherhouse or the bishop to begin a novitiate of their own, Lawrencetta did what they had always done in Mokama: she improvised and made the best of what she had. She decided to accept Bridget and the others in that first group as students, two for nursing and three for the pharmacy training institute led by Crescentia. Informally, they were told they would eventually become nuns.

It was a confusing arrangement for everyone. The first batch of Indian postulants—Bridget's class—stayed in the same dormitory as the nursing students. Bridget and the other candidates reluctantly accepted the situation. If entering the order meant getting medical training as well, they couldn't see the harm in it; they did not necessarily want to be nurses or pharmacists, but if that's what it took to become part of the order, they were willing to do it.

The student nurses, on the other hand, knew why they were there and had begun to form a tight community. They had no interest in religious life; they were there for the training and the opportunities it might open. By 1955, when Bridget entered, there were enough student nurses, some from the north and some from Kerala, to staff three shifts in the hospital. Some had been in Mokama long enough to have done their specialized training in midwifery and had started to work as staff nurses. They didn't understand what Bridget and the others were doing there. Why would anyone come all the way to Bihar to join an order of American nuns when there were orders of Indian women much closer to home in Kerala? If they were really going to become full-fledged members of the Sisters of Charity of Nazareth, one of the nurses asked Bridget, why weren't they given quarters with the American sisters? Why were they being told to study anatomy instead of canon law? They warned Bridget, "They will mistreat you. They will treat you like second-class citizens."

The first few weeks were hard. Bridget wanted to be a nun right away, but instead she was sitting in class studying nursing. She had not even been given a choice—the priest had arbitrarily assigned her to nursing instead of pharmacy training. She hated it. She hated the dirt and brown dust that seemed to be everywhere in Mokama; it was nothing like the cool green grass and coconut palms of Meenachil. And what was she learning? As far as Bridget could tell, nursing was mostly cleaning. She learned to wash the windows, swab the floors, and wipe down the metal beds after each patient was discharged.

She had never been exposed to the level of poverty that people in Mokama endured. In Kerala, there were poor people, of course. But nearly every child went to school and had something to eat, and bathing was as simple as walking down to the nearest creek. Here, she spent her days in the wards, with the patients' families crowded anxiously around their beds. They seeemed to have no education, and they had only one set of clothes that they wore all day and slept in. The smell nauseated Bridget. For a month, she felt she could hardly eat.

Even worse, Lawrencetta seemed to have rejected her. Soon after Bridget arrived, Lawrencetta introduced the five would-be nuns in Bridget's group to a visiting parish priest. "These are the four who are joining us." She didn't include Bridget, indicating that she had come only to study nursing. The slight tormented Bridget. Why did Lawrencetta exclude her? For what other reason did she think she had left her home, with no way to return? Certainly not for the drudgery of being a nursing student. She would fall asleep in tears, trying to understand what had happened. But she did not have enough English to express her confusion and frustration to those forbidding American women, and she had nowhere else to turn.

After a few weeks, when she had grown more confident in English, Bridget put the words together. "Why are you not considering me a candidate?" she asked. Lawrencetta explained to her calmly that the priest who had arranged her passage to Mokama told the nuns it was Bridget's wish. Immediately, Bridget wrote an angry letter to the priest in Kerala—"Why did you do that?"—and waited for his reply. The priest admitted to the deception; he wrote to her that he had done so at the instruction of Bridget's father, who was not ready to part with her. He could not accept that his daughter, with all the privileges he had given her, had chosen the hard life of the convent over the future he imagined, of education, comfort, and success. He had agreed, reluctantly, to allow her to go, but he wanted her to come home every year during Christmas like any other student. So he had secretly made an agreement with the priest. Bridget was furious. She put down the letter from the priest and wrote to her father: "I will never come home again."

In that year, 1955, unrest of many kinds rumbled through Indian society. In May, in Kanpur, a few hundred miles upstream from Mokama, 46,000 textile workers went on strike to protest the modernization of some of the mills, in a city where tanneries just a decade earlier had produced boots for the British Army. The strike lasted more than two months—the longest at the time in the history of Indian trade unions. Workers in Bombay had similar grievances, but the labor action they began in August took on an additional political texture: they had claimed as their own the cause of independence for Goa. The Portuguese territory on the southwestern coast was one of the last vestiges of the colonial past, and Goans were clamoring for India to intercede on their behalf. More than 150,000 textile mill workers, shop clerks, railway workers, and dock hands joined a general strike in support of the Goan liberation movement.

Portugal had troops in Goa, and the situation quickly escalated. A protest against a shooting by Portuguese troops of people at the border prompted a call by India's leftist parties for a nationwide general strike. By August 17, Calcutta was all but shut down. That August, a month after Bridget arrived, the Annals recorded the arrival of a sister who came to stay with them, possibly for months, so she could study for her nursing exams. Her school was one of many that had been closed because of the uprising of the students against the government. The schools remained closed for two weeks.

Estranged from her family, Bridget resolved to stay in Mokama. She would have to find a way to remain at the convent on her own terms. She began to talk with the four others who had come with her to be candidates. They considered their options. Maybe they wouldn't join the order at all. What if the student nurses were right and the American women started to treat them badly? They could stay just long enough to finish their courses and get their training, and then go home.

The weeks passed, and nothing terrible happened; the sisters treated them just as they did the other students. So Bridget and the others decided to stay. For more than a year, the would-be novices studied with the nurses, and in 1956, Bridget and the others all passed their first-year nursing exams. But there was no sign that the order was taking any steps to welcome them as candidates for the novitiate; they weren't even given any extra religious obligations. All the young women were expected to go to Mass every day. Bridget was impatient for something to change.

She didn't know it then, but there was a reason for the delay. Lawrencetta had already made an application to open a novitiate, and she knew there were plenty of women interested in joining them. "So we know the vocations will come as soon as we open the doors," she wrote. But Mother Bertrand told her to wait. A novitiate was not yet part of their plan. It was enough of a financial and organizational challenge for them to support the work of a hospital and nursing school in Mokama and a school in Gaya. Were they really ready to handle a novitiate as well?

Mother Bertrand asked the vicar general of the Diocese of Patna for advice, and he told her that the order should wait until they had been in India for at least ten years before even thinking about a novitiate. So Mother Bertrand decided that they could begin in 1957.

The news was disappointing, but Lawrencetta accepted the decision. In any case, they did not have enough professed sisters to run the hospital and supervise a group of novices. "We need some recruits before we can spare a sister to take charge of the novitiate," she wrote to her family. Besides, the convent was short on space; Lawrencetta felt that their novitiate in Mokama should be just like the one in Kentucky, where the sisters in training were kept apart, physically and spiritually, from everyone else, the better to focus on the discernment of their vocation. So in May 1956, she started work on expanding the chapel so that they would have a separate dormitory for the novices before the new novitiate building was ready.

Bridget wasn't told about any of these deliberations or quiet changes. After a year of waiting, she and the others said to one another that the sisters were not doing anything to bring them into the congregation. They knew there were women in the nursing school who were members of other religious orders, and therefore given the honor of special visits by their director. It was a small gesture, but it signaled to the other students that those girls were special: they belonged somewhere other than the nursing school. But Bridget felt that she and the other four were just being lumped in with everyone else. Soon after passing their exams, they decided to do something.

On the first day of their protest, they refused to go to Mass. No one said anything. On the second day, when they again did not turn up at Mass, Florence Joseph came up to them in a fury to find out what was going on. "What happened?" she asked. Bridget replied calmly, "We are on strike. Because you are not doing anything to make us candidates." She told Florence Joseph that the five of them resented the way they were being treated and wanted to feel that they were part of the order—not simply nursing students passing through on the way to somewhere else.

Florence Joseph was incredulous. A strike? This kind of overt disobedience was unheard of in the Sisters of Charity of Nazareth. She immediately went to Lawrencetta, who took it in stride. "Well, I'll write to Mother Bertrand and find out what we can do." This time, Lawrencetta didn't wait for a reply from the motherhouse. She asked Crescentia to start leading a Sunday-morning instruction class for the candidates to make it clear that they were on a special path. Bridget knew she had won.

Lawrencetta, who would be in charge of the postulants' guidance and spiritual formation, made her first recruiting trip as newly appointed mistress of novices in December 1956, right after Christmas, with an ambitious plan to fly to Bombay, Mangalore, and then Cochin, the centers of traditional Catholic life in India. She expected to find so many prospects—novices but perhaps nursing students as well—that she would have to bring them back to Mokama by rail.

She and Eugenia, part of the new batch of Kentucky sisters, arrived at six in the morning in Bombay, where they met the bishop of Nagpur and stayed at Villa Theresa, the same place where the sisters on the *Steel Executive* had briefly stopped when they first landed in India. Lawrencetta met several priests, who promised to send recruits, and spent a similar day in Mangalore.

Cochin, the storied port on the Kerala coast, was completely different. The landscape was unlike anything she had ever seen before. There were so many canals and streams, the backwaters of Kerala, that she wasn't sure where their plane might land. There seemed to be more water than earth. And the people she met were not the cosmopolitan Catholics of Bombay; she needed an interpreter everywhere she went to translate her American English and the Malayalam spoken in Kerala. Lawrencetta's hard-won Hindi was useless here.

Slowly, over the next two weeks, Lawrencetta and Eugenia made their way inland, farther and farther by bus into smaller and smaller towns in the Catholic heartland of Kerala. Lawrencetta was amazed by the number and persistence of the young women who came to see them. "All week long the girls kept coming in, making application, some for nurses training and some for the novitiate." Still, she was skeptical. "Their English is so poor, that they will have to have special studies in this for about six months or so, before they will understand us freely." High schools in Kerala taught in Malayalam, with only one period of English. The girls were seldom able to understand what she was saying, but they were undeterred.

And they were so young. "One day a little girl came in, only fifteen years of age and small for that." She had come with a letter from her pastor, saying that ever since she had seen the notice in the paper, she had given him no peace and insisted that he write her a letter of support. Lawrencetta was dismissive. Even if the girl had a true vocation, she thought, she would have to grow up a little bit more or try an order closer to home.

Was this really the answer to Nazareth Hospital's nursing shortage? They seemed eager, but they weren't prepared. Lawrencetta brought back only two candidates and a few nursing students. She wanted to wait and see whether these vocations held up over time, whether these delicate young women could persevere through the hardships of life in Mokama and the isolation of life in a convent.

On her last night in Champakulam, before she went on to Palai to see one of the priests who had already sent several recruits, Lawrencetta visited the women of a "native order," the Convent of the Blessed Sacrament Sisters. She could barely communicate with them, but after nearly two weeks in Kerala it hardly seemed to matter. It was getting dark, and one of the sisters asked Lawrecentta "if she had had her bath for the day." When she replied that she had not, the sister suggested, "Probably you would like to take it now. We bathe in the river."

They led her to the concrete bathhouse built into the riverbank—"two rooms about ten feet square, with steps leading down to the water." Lawrencetta hesitated; she didn't know how to swim and she was embarrassed about the possibility of someone catching a glimpse of her bathing. "I had visions of myself going in the river and said maybe we had [better] wait until it was darker." But as the light faded over the jade green water, Lawrencetta's fears released their hold on her. She stood in the bathhouse and carefully removed her pleated bonnet, the stiff cotton habit, and then her socks. Traditionally, the habit included stockings, but these had become almost impossible to find when import controls were imposed, especially those large enough for her size 10½ feet.

The first two steps were above water, and as she stepped farther down, the water became deeper and she immersed herself in the river, the same backwaters that channeled through the villages where Bridget and Rose had grown up, through the same red earth that had once stained their feet and the hems of their skirts. "The water was much warmer than what we are accustomed to," Lawrencetta wrote, "and I was agreeably surprised and thoroughly enjoyed the bath."

Upon her return to Mokama, Lawrencetta took Crescentia's advice and interpreted Mother Bertrand's decision about the beginning of the order as liberally as possible. If they were allowed, according to the bishop's instructions, to begin their novitiate in 1957, why not "begin" by retroactively bringing into the fold the five women who had already been there for two years? They opened the novitiate on February 2.

Bridget began the regimented life of a sister in training. She would wake up at 5:00, pray and meditate with the group at 5:30, then attend Mass at 6:30. After Mass, they all had breakfast in the hospital kitchen, usually bread, butter, and jam. When they were not working in the hospital, they were assigned to clean the novitiate, the name for the space that the five of them occupied at one end of the second floor, and wash their clothes. (The dhobi washed only the sisters' habits.) After another hour of prayer, they began their classes—usually two or three of them a day. Lawrencetta taught some of them; the priest took others. There was theology, Scripture, English, the history of the order, its constitution, and Church history. Later, when they resumed their nursing classes, they had one or two classes a day at the hospital with the student nurses.

Lawrencetta was a natural in her new role as mistress of novices—methodical and prayerful, calm and orderly. Her goal was to maintain the heritage of the congregation, to convey to these young women from Kerala the history and traditions of a community that they had never seen. She wanted them to understand—especially after that painful misunderstanding in their first year—that they were fully a part of this religious community, not foreign or secondary in any way. So she tried to create a cocoon for them, a place set apart from the world of the hospital. She understood that they were young women and needed time to themselves. During the day, from noon to three, the candidates had to observe "sacred silence," remaining silent unless absolute necessary, but in the evenings, between tea and evening prayers, she encouraged them to play volleyball or badminton on the wide lawns outside, near the shrine.

After supper, Lawrencetta would join Bridget and the others for "common recreation." They would bring their mending, sit and sew, and talk about whatever amusing things had happened during the day. Lawrencetta encouraged them to laugh and speak freely, and after a few months, their English was confident enough that it felt more natural to talk to one another in English. Lawrencetta was warm, but didn't reveal much of herself to the candidates. Bridget knew that Lawrencetta had two unmarried sisters, who were great supporters of the mission in Mokama. She did not tell them about the third, who had died suddenly after their mother passed away. Or another sister, who was a nun with another order but suffered from mental illness and spent the last years of her life in and out of touch with reality. But the young novices wrote condolence letters to her family after the death of her brother Lawrence. They learned bits and pieces of her life before Mokama: that she knew the constellations and could dance the Virginia reel. That she loved music and had been a music teacher, and would play the piano for them in church. She assigned them a whimsical chore: when the bright sun began to burn through the early spring sky, the novices and postulants gathered around a large cotton tree on the campus to pluck the soft bunches of fiber, tossing them into the air with delight before gathering them to use as stuffing for pillows. Later, on one special Christmas morning, she allowed the novices to sleep in and woke them up gently to the sound of her violin playing as another sister sang, "Awake O Slumbering World."

By the end of 1957, Bridget became one of the first Indian women to receive her habit as a member of the Sisters of Charity of Nazareth. She was excited to finally take this step. She would be set apart, no longer bound by the world she had been born into. To prepare herself, on the night before the ceremony, she wrote down three names, one of which would become hers: "Ann Philip" (the names of her mother and father, one of the most common naming conventions in the order); "Ann Joseph" (her mother and grandfather); and "Joseph Maria" (her brother and oldest sister). She didn't know which one the senior sisters would choose for her.

Then Bridget submitted to a ritual required of all the new sisters.

Lawrencetta told Bridget to tie her long, thick hair in two tight braids. They went to the common room and took turns, according to age, sitting in the chair that had been placed there. Bridget was the youngest of the group, so she went last. She cried as she felt the weight of the scissors separating the glossy plaits from her body. "Here it is," Lawrencetta said. Bridget took the hair and later sent it home, so one of her sisters could use it as a "fall," or hairpiece, for formal occasions.

The next morning, she was again called to the common room to be given her new white habit, which had been blessed by the priests. She went to her room, dressed, and came back to receive her new name. Bridget became "Ann Philip," although neither of her parents attended the Mass in their honor later that day. It would be nine years before she saw them again, but one relative, a brother-in-law, came to Mokama for the ceremony, to represent the family. When the Mass was over, she went back to her quarters and discarded everything she owned that had her old name written on it.

FOURTEEN

The English-Only Rule

O nce the novitiate was established, the student nurses occupied a separate world bound by its own set of rules. Their lives at Mokama were contained on three floors of one building: the hospital taking up most of the first floor, the chapel and classrooms on the second, and the nurses' hostel and dining hall on the third.

For Rose, after the relative freedom of her life in Palai, life in Mokama was a shock. The constant stream of admonitions from the nuns—you have to do this, you have to do that—began almost the moment she reached Mokama. The sisters believed that head lice and tapeworms were endemic in India, and they did not want them to take hold in the hospital, so every nurse had to endure an application of DDT in her hair and medication for worms within a few days after arriving.

Like Bridget, Rose found it difficult to understand what the sisters said. They were all so big and imposing, and she would sometimes sit and look at them in awe, these strange, pale creatures, their accents forming words that seemed familiar and yet sounded like nothing she had ever heard before. For the first six months, she sat for an hour of English lessons every day at 11:00 a.m. It was sometimes hard to concentrate on the lesson because she was thinking about what to say if the sisters asked her a question. She learned that you must always greet a sister when she passed. "Good morning, sister." If she seemed to be asking a question or making a request, the correct response was usually "Thank you, sister." From the tone, she could sometimes guess that it might also be "Yes, sister" or "No, sister." She was too scared to listen to what they were actually saying.

There wasn't enough room in the dining hall for all the student nurses to eat at the same time, so they would take turns and go class by class, the senior classes first. Rose had to wait for the older girls to finish their meal before she could begin, each group washing the dishes of the one that ate before them. The sisters taught them the rules for the proper "American" way to wash dishes: there were three dishpans full of water, one for dirty plates to remove the food, another with soapy water to clean them, and a third with fresh water to rinse them.

In the evenings, Rose went to the veranda, where the newest girls had their beds because there wasn't enough room for all of them to sleep indoors in the dormitory—the sisters were slowly building a new addition to the nursing school. She sat with the others and talked in Malayalam, taking refuge in the language she had spoken at home, the language that reminded her of the sound of rough, dried grains of rice being shaken and tossed in a wide basket to remove the hulls.

She was never alone. Mokama was full of girls like her, those who needed something more than what they would find in Kerala. Leela had come to Mokama a few years before Rose did, when she was only sixteen. She had a cousin who was a nun in Bettiah who had told her about the sisters' work in Mokama. Her older sister was working as a nurse in a government hospital in Kerala, but Leela wanted something more. Her father didn't think she would survive in a nursing school run by nuns. "How are you going to put up with it?" he had asked her. "You argue over everything."

There was Elizabeth, the schoolteacher's daughter. Her parents had doted on her—music lessons, drama lessons, two new frilly dresses from the tailor every season. Elizabeth was a good student, so when a girls' college opened in Kottayam, her father wanted her to go there. But on the day she was sent by bus to register for classes, with her cash deposit and high school certificate in her purse, Elizabeth simply refused to go. She got off the bus, went to her grandparents' house instead, and then turned around and came back. She wanted to be a nun, like so many of her friends, or work as a nurse in an army hospital like the one her family had once visited in Kerala's new capital. She had thirty days before she would lose her place at the college, and soon learned that the army hospitals wouldn't take her—she was too young. Her father found a sympathetic priest who arranged for her to join a group heading to Mokama.

And there was Elsy, one of the girls who had traveled with Rose to Mokama and became one of her closest friends. She had grown up in a village called Pravithanam, full of rubber and teak plantations and not much else. Elsy, too, had grown up without a father. He had abandoned their family when Elsy was a baby. He left Elsy's mother with two daughters, a few acres of rubber trees, and the taint of scandal. Because their household didn't have a man, her mother needed someone to help her take care of the property, to take on the role of "duth nikhyan," the man who moves into his wife's house and accepts her family's property and obligations. In the traditional arrangement, the wife was an asset, acquired by the husband's family to bear children and help take care of the husband's property and family. People in Kerala looked down on such men, so it took some time before her mother could find someone to agree to a match. Her older sister married at seventeen. This sacrifice freed Elsy, who was then fifteen, but she had to make a choice. She could either find a husband, someone willing to accept a girl from a broken family, or she could leave.

She had few models for how leaving might be done. All the women in Pravithanam stayed at home; even the teachers were all men. There were movie stars—the three Travancore sisters who sang and danced in the Malayalam films she loved to watch in the cinema hall in Palai, and Miss Kumari, who had gone to Catholic school in Bharananganam and somehow became a film star, something she thought only Hindus did. A few of the girls who were good at math went on to become college professors or teachers. Rich girls went to college to study "home science" and learn the fashionable new ways of cooking, baking, and sewing, and would usually be married or at least engaged by the time they finished college. Elsy was terrible at math, and she wasn't rich. The only other profession she had actually heard of for women was nursing. She had seen them in the clinic nearby. They seemed so timid, just doing what the doctors told them to do. They must have had some training, but if they had a real degree, surely they wouldn't have been working in a small place like that.

She had heard about nursing schools in Nagpur, Delhi, Vellore, Bombay, and Jamshedpur. But her mother would never allow her to go to a city where they didn't know anyone. Two of her cousins had gone to North India somewhere. When they came back for their first vacation, they were speaking English and they talked about the American nuns who were teaching them. That's what she wanted, to study with Americans and become a "real" nurse, like them. Her mother didn't object; she talked to the priest, and Elsy, too, made her way to Mokama.

The nuns wouldn't allow them to leave the compound unchaperoned, so what else was there to do in Mokama but talk? They were teenagers, and they found it difficult to put aside their disgust at the dirt and stench from the very sick and very poor patients who filled the beds at Nazareth Hospital. The patients suffered from misfortunes they had never seen or heard of in Kerala. There was leprosy and tuberculosis, of course, and the fevers that claimed so many children all over India. But there were also snakebites and a constant stream of knife injuries—casualties of the caste wars that were starting to roll across Bihar. And the abortions that had gone horribly wrong, when women who had inserted chewing tobacco into their vaginas, hoping to induce a miscarriage, ended up in the hospital with sepsis. Rose and the others lay on the thin mattresses they had brought with them in their trunks, trying to make sense of it all, spooling out the night hours on their cots, next to women who could have been their sisters or aunts or cousins, just as they did at home.

They tried to model themselves on the example of the American sisters, who had devoted themselves to the poor of Mokama for years without complaint. But it was Celine Minj, who had become a supervisor at Nazareth nine months after she was named a staff nurse, who showed them exactly what to do and how to survive. The essential but unpleasant work of keeping the patients and everything else in the hospital clean fell primarily to the nursing students: sterilizing instruments, mopping floors, cleaning windows, emptying bedpans, cleaning bloody and soiled linens after deliveries, disinfecting the beds, and airing the mattresses in the sun. She explained how to get their uniforms washed by the dhobi. Each of the nurses were given four-teen uniforms—seven to wash and seven to wear. There were so many new nurses arriving that the newest ones had to make do with fewer until the tailor could catch up.

Celine had been doing this for various nurses in training since the earliest days of the hospital. In the years before there was piped water, Celine demonstrated how to carry the bucket from the well in the middle of the courtyard up the stairs to their rooms on the third floor. Before the power lines reached Mokama, she escorted the nurses to the generator shed and told them to find the mistry to turn it on. Rose and the others had it easy in comparison, Celine told them. But when the electricity failed, she taught them how to make their rounds by lantern light, with one hand free and the other on the lantern so they could somehow still see what they were doing.

Once they had some basic training, the young nurses were as-signed to the night shifts, 11:00 p.m. to 7:00 a.m., and Celine showed them how to manage. When the shift began, the day nurse would give them charges—the instructions for each patient and what they would require overnight. Every patient needed something, so the nurses would make the rounds to all the beds and make notes in their charts along the way. Some had IVs for dehydration; some had diarrhea, so they would call for bedpans. Some of them were women in labor. Every pregnant woman who arrived at Nazareth Hospital was as-signed to a different nurse, who would see the woman through the delivery, with Celine's help. But when their labor continued for hours into the night, as it often did, the student on night duty would have to keep watch and know when to call Celine and the assigned nurse for the delivery, and when to call the doctor for complications.

For the nurses who arrived in the summer, as Rose and most of the others did, the beginning of winter a few months later brought yet

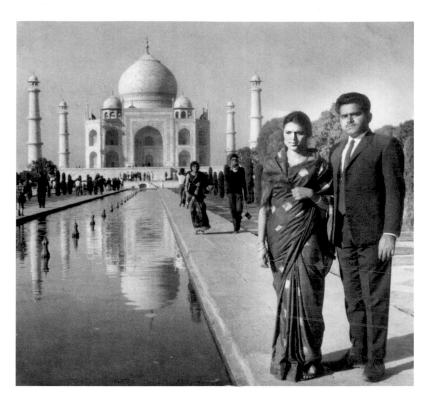

Author's parents at the Taj Mahal, February 1971.

Courtesy of the author

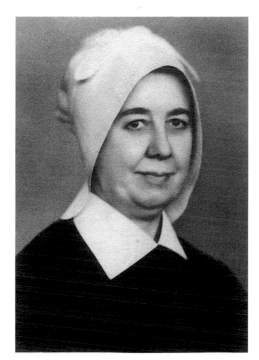

An undated photo of
Mother Ann Sebastian
Sullivan, who made the
decision to begin the order's
first mission overseas.

*Courtesy of Sisters of Charity
of Nazareth Archival Center*

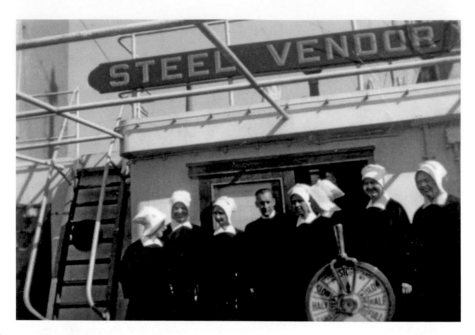

A group of well-wishers, including other members of the order, gathered to send off Sisters Lawrencetta, Ann Cornelius, and Crescentia on the *Steel Vendor*.

Courtesy of Sisters of Charity of Nazareth Archival Center

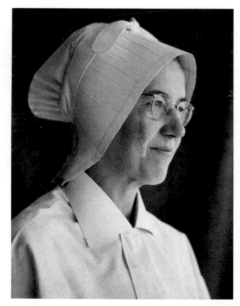

Undated photo of Sister Lawrencetta Veeneman, the first leader of the mission at Nazareth Hospital.

Courtesy of the Veeneman family

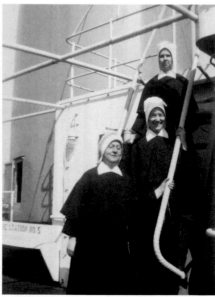

(left to right) Sisters Crescentia Wise, Lawrencetta Veeneman, and Ann Cornelius Curran on the *Steel Vendor* in 1947, on their way to India.

Courtesy of the Veeneman family

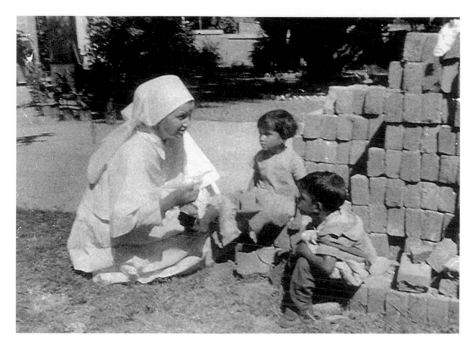

Sister Ann Roberta, the youngest of the six pioneers, with children in Bihar.
Her ease with Hindi made her a favorite among the people of Mokama.

Courtesy of Sisters of Charity of Nazareth Archival Center

Sisters Charles Miriam,
Lawrencetta, and Ann
Roberta look up at Sisters
Ann Cornelius and
Crescentia as they ride an
elephant owned by one
of Mokama's wealthy
landowning families,
in an undated photo on
the grounds of Nazareth
Hospital. Elephant rides
were a popular subject
for photos sent home to
Kentucky.

*Courtesy of Sisters of Charity of
Nazareth Archival Center*

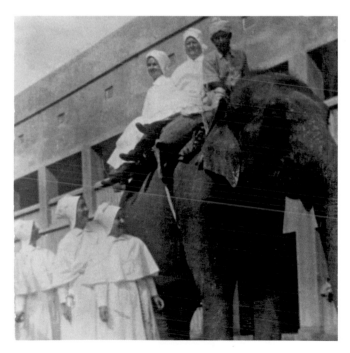

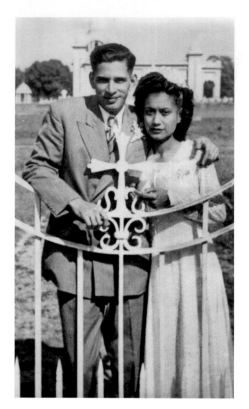

Dr. Eric Lazaro, Nazareth
Hospital's first doctor, and
Babs Gillard on the day of their
wedding, in front of the shrine
at Mokama, December 1949.

Courtesy of Erica Lazaro

A cycle rickshaw
driver with
Sisters Ann
Roberta Powers
(left, standing)
and Charles
Miriam Holt
(right, seated)
at Nazareth
Academy in Gaya.
The two sisters
left Mokama at
the end of 1950
to take over the
leadership of the
school.

*Courtesy of Sisters of
Charity of Nazareth
Archival Center*

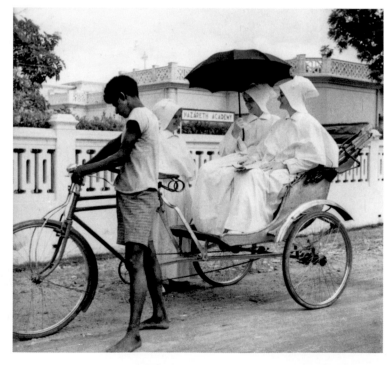

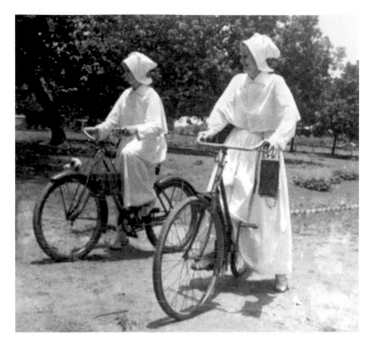

Sisters Ann Cornelius Curran and Florence Joseph Sauer,
in an undated photo, riding the bicycles that the order acquired
to get around the hospital campus efficiently.

Courtesy of Sisters of Charity of Nazareth Archival Center

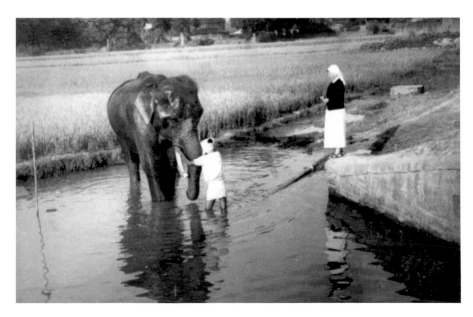

Sister Ann Roberta in Bihar, in an undated photo.

Courtesy of Sisters of Charity of Nazareth Archival Center

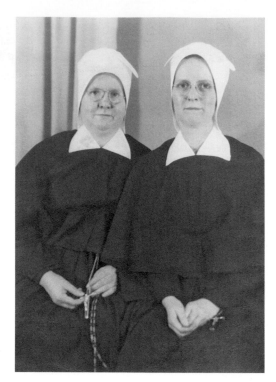

Sister Crescentia Wise *(left)*, with her sister, Willie Mae Wise, known as Sister Ellen Mary, on July 4, 1947.

Courtesy of Dolores Vittitow

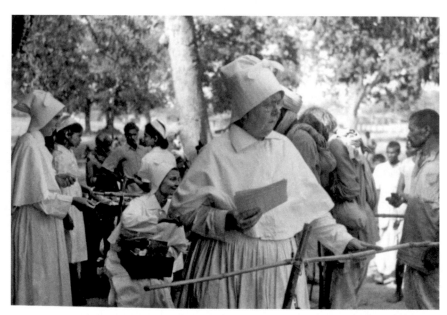

In an undated photo, Sister Crescentia Wise oversees the large group of Hansen's disease patients gathered at Nazareth Hospital for the weekly clinic. The bamboo poles were an improvised method of keeping order.

Courtesy of Sisters of Charity of Nazareth Archival Center

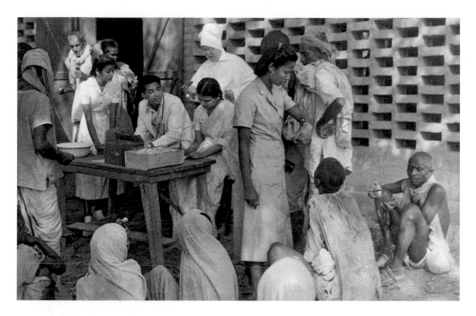

Sister Crescentia Wise (in white habit) with a doctor and hospital staff registering patients for the Hansen's disease clinic. The clinic registered thousands of patients, managing their biweekly doses of diasone, a drug that stopped the progress of leprosy.

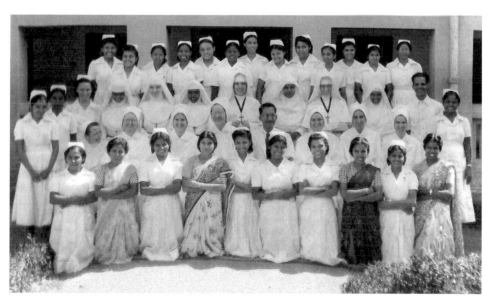

Members of the faculty and student body of the newly opened school of nursing at Nazareth Hospital in Mokama in October 1953. The students are a mix of Indian women and nuns from other orders (pictured in full white veils and wimples, distinct from the sunbonnets worn by the Sisters of Charity of Nazareth).

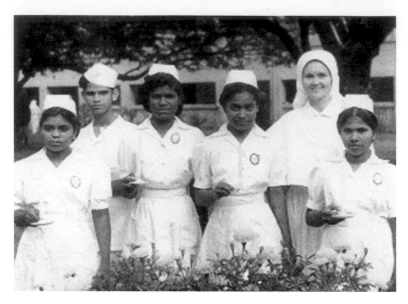

Sister Florence Joseph Sauer (in habit) with five new nurses in 1956,
including Bridget Kappalumakal, third from right.

Courtesy of Sisters of Charity of Nazareth Archival Center

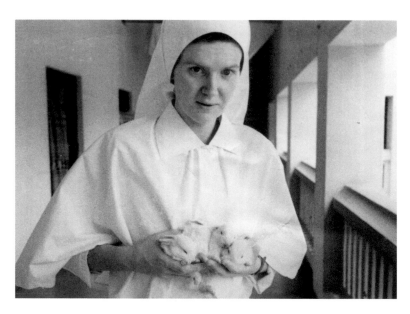

Mary Martha Wiss in July 1960 in Mokama. She wrote on the
back of the photo: "This is me and the baby rabbits."

Courtesy of the Wiss family

another kind of silent suffering. There was nothing like this cold in Kerala, where even the winters were warm and mild. The nurses learned to wear two sets of gloves, coats, then a cap. Night duty was particularly horrible, as the temperature overnight hovered just above freezing. The nurses were supposed to wash their hands after touching anything, and even after the hospital got piped water, it was not heated. In the winter, it was like pouring ice water over your fingers. They never warmed up; the girls simply had to wait until morning, sleep as long as they could, and warm their hands in the sun the next day. Rose learned that if she was very lucky, all the patients would fall asleep at some point during the night—but it was rare for them all to do so at once. If there was a spare moment, Celine told her, you can rest in a chair and sit down, but you can never sleep.

Instead of Lawrencetta, whose presence faded from the hospital as she spent most of her time with the novices, the student nurses became the wards of Sister Florence Joseph, who had taken over the running of the school. Born Mary Frances Sauer, Florence Joseph had grown up on a farm in Smith Mills in western Kentucky, on the Ohio River about eighty miles west of Cloverport, where Ann Roberta was born. Florence Joseph was different from calm, measured Lawrencetta and had none of her ponderousness. While Lawrencetta had grown up in a grand house in Louisville, with a keen sense of living up to the Veenemans' position among the established Catholic families of the city, Florence Joseph was a farmer's daughter. Both of her parents came from German immigrant families who had settled in southern Indiana in the late 1800s. They were born in Evansville, Indiana, and crossed the Ohio River to settle in Kentucky shortly after they married. They raised seven children—two girls and five boys—on their farm, with the help of a laborer who lived in their rented house as a boarder.

Florence Joseph had no particular family tradition to continue or status to maintain; her life was hers to make of it what she could. She joined the convent at the age of nineteen in 1938, received her habit in 1939, and took her first vows on March 25, 1940, the day before she started her training as a nurse at Saints Mary and Elizabeth Hospital in Louisville. (By that point, two of her brothers were still on the farm, old enough to take on the labor themselves.) She spent the war years as a nurse at nearby Mt. Saint Agnes, and was still there in 1947 when the mission to India began.

A generation younger than Lawrencetta, Florence Joseph was only thirty-seven years old when she took over as superior for the hospital and nursing school. While Lawrencetta wrote letters and made methodical plans to get Nazareth Hospital through its first decade, Florence Joseph raced into the second decade with grand ideas that seemed to materialize on the spot. Her voice carried, whether raised in delight or anger, and she would walk through the compound, her long limbs gesticulating wildly, saying, we need a building here, we need this there. She seemed open to every new idea that passed through the air.

She once went to a ten-day meeting in Calcutta on the subject of "Psychological Counseling and Guidance in India." It was conducted by a Spanish Jesuit, a psychologist who had spent several years as a counselor in Bombay and was trying to popularize the idea of mental health and counseling as an ordinary part of the services offered by schools and hospitals. He encouraged the sisters to include psychological care to new candidates as part of the discernment process. About ninety sisters from various orders in Calcutta attended, and not all of them were convinced. Mother Teresa, for example, attended but felt that psychological counseling struck her as a "Western" concept, and decided that she and her order would continue to work with the skills they already had. But Florence Joseph immediately thought, "Yes, we should do this." She was open to this new idea, and it would prove especially important in the subsequent years, as women in religious communities had to grapple with profound changes in the Catholic Church and their role within it.

Florence Joseph understood that they were in India to do big things and should sometimes move forward even if the path was unclear. And she found creative ways to get things done. Going beyond the order's usual sources of funds, from the parishes the order served in Kentucky and the surrounding states, she raised thousands of rupees from donors in the United States, India, and Germany for a new isolation wing and a separate novitiate building, both of which eventually eased the overcrowding in the hospital.

To the student nurses, Florence Joseph seemed temperamental and sometimes unreasonably strict. Everything had to be perfect, from the cleanliness of the floors to the way the nurses handled the patients. Mattresses had to be aired out in the sunlight. Windows had to be washed. The beds had to be disinfected every time a patient left. While Lawrencetta was motherly, gentle even in her scolding, Florence Joseph was always moving, always watching, the type of supervisor who would literally run her finger across a table or bed frame to check for dust.

The young nurses rarely saw the sisters outside the hospital or the classroom; in the evenings, they would see the American women walking to prayers and off to the convent. But they learned to be wary. Florence Joseph would sometimes send one of the other sisters to patrol the dormitory, unannounced, looking for rule breakers. They weren't supposed to walk holding hands with the other girls or with their hands on each other's shoulders. They were never to sleep in each other's beds, as they often did at home. The girls knew little about sex or lesbian relationships, but they knew enough to understand that the sisters were suspicious of any close friendship or displays of affection among the students. Above all, they were never to be heard speaking Malayalam. The young nurses knew the sisters were coming because they could hear the swish and click of their rosary beads as they walked. When the sound suddenly stopped, they knew one of the sisters must be close by and had clutched the rosary in her hand to silence it.

The young nurses were all so homesick, especially for rice. They grew up eating rice twice a day and found it difficult to have chapatis for lunch and dinner. The student nurses noticed that the novices had started to eat separately, and often had rice. The nuns seemed to treat them a little better; they had committed their lives to the order and had been taken into the fold of the convent. So the nurses would steal rice, just to give their bellies that familiar sensation and be able to rest. They felt guilty, of course. So they would tally up their crimes and recount them in letters to the chaplain, Father Ziebert, or tell him in confession. And he would give them absolution. If you're hungry, and you take something to eat, it's all right, he told them. He knew how hard it was for them to be so far away from their families; he was American, and even farther from home.

When the young nurses inevitably fell short of Florence Joseph's standards, she would lose her temper and then just as quickly forget it had ever happened. One day, Leela finally had enough. Sitting wearily at the dining table after a particularly difficult night shift, she waited for a morning meal to sustain her through a few hours of rest and the next day's classes. But instead of the usual rice and curry, the kitchen boy handed her a plate of tea biscuits. Leela crushed the biscuits in anger and went to Florence Joseph to complain. "Honey, would you behave like this at home?" the sister asked her. When Florence Joseph called the nurses "honey," they knew she was angry. But Leela didn't care. She snapped back at her, "At home, they won't keep me starving like this." Sometimes, the best way to deal with Florence Joseph was to give as good as you got.

Florence Joseph also pushed the nurses to do more than they ever thought possible. When she saw how many women struggled on the long journey through the village roads around Mokama to the hospital to deliver their babies, she started sending the student nurses out in pairs to conduct prenatal checkups and deliveries. Never mind that none of them had any real experience with sex or childbirth; they went armed with whatever they had learned in class. Rose and her partner, at their first delivery, couldn't find the words to tell the laboring mother to lie down on the mud floor, as the textbooks had instructed. The mother just looked at them, squatted on a brick, and delivered the baby without any help from the two young nurses, who could do nothing but giggle with embarrassment.

Occasionally, Florence Joseph had the capacity to laugh at herself, as she did when her gangly frame sometimes got the better of her. The annals record one notorious afternoon in which she took all the lay nurses for a picnic and somehow got too close to a wandering cow, which knocked her into a ditch. "In falling she pulled one of the nurses after her and but for the quick work of Father Rodriguez the nurse would have fallen into the river."

Once they learned how to handle Florence Joseph's moods, the young nurses started to enjoy working in the hospital. Each of the sisters was a little different. Ann Cornelius was the stickler in the operating room. That was her domain, and it sometimes seemed as if she never left it. Being an operating-room nurse was different from working in the general wards. It wasn't about warmth or patient care or diagnosing a complicated set of symptoms. Working in the OR required precision and speed and absolute focus. Not every nurse was suited to this work, and Ann Cornelius had her favorites, like Leela, who had a certain toughness that suited surgical nursing. Leela liked the challenge and rigor of the operating room, and Ann Cornelius would ask for her, in particular, any time there was a special case, like a complicated delivery. The other nurses resented Ann Cornelius's favorites; everyone else would be left with the thankless task of cleaning up afterward.

Working in the pharmacy with Crescentia was more fun. The area set aside as the pharmacy wasn't much—a simple room, shelves, an almirah, and lots of medicine bottles. The nurses would register the patients and record the prices paid for the vitamins and antibiotics, and the medicines for diarrhea, fever, pain, headache, skin diseases, and leprosy. They kept the medicines for emergencies—like the antidotes for snakebites—in the almirah so they could get to them easily. The students all knew Crescentia was a heart patient who had high blood pressure, but nothing seemed to slow her down. She was there in the pharmacy every morning at 7:30 and stayed until 6:00 in the evening when it closed. Crescentia was also the one sister who didn't seem to mind when they poked fun, at her clumsy Hindi and at the strange figure she cut in Mokama.

One incident became legendary among the nurses—when Crescentia, heroine of the leprosy clinic, offered a young man her umbrella, her "chahtha," as protection against the punishing sun, as he left the hospital to go out to a village to meet a leprosy patient. But

Crescentia instead offered him her "chahthi," her breast, generating a roar of embarrassed laughter from the crowd.

The one rule that the young nurses could not abide was Florence Joseph's insistence on speaking English. The American sisters had spent so many difficult months learning Hindi, thinking it would bring them closer to the people of India. And yet here was a group of Indian women speaking a completely different language, unrelated to both Hindi and English. The sisters taught nursing classes in English—their Hindi wasn't good enough to teach anatomy and nursing procedure in it—but they expected that the young nurses would have arrived with enough Hindi to manage communicating with the patients on their own and enough English to understand the sisters' instructions. Nazareth Hospital would only accept girls who had high school diplomas and therefore had, in theory, earned passing grades in Hindi and English, both of which were required subjects. Instead, the girls struggled to turn their rote knowledge of Hindi into useful conversations with patients or to speak English well enough to talk freely with the sisters. So Florence Joseph and the other sisters made it clear that the student nurses would be punished if they were ever caught speaking Malayalam, even to one another.

It may have seemed like a necessary, if extreme, measure to ensure that nurses trained at Nazareth Hospital would have skills to match those of the best nurses in India. But the English-only rule collided with one of the most sensitive issues in the first two decades of free India—language.

By 1955, language had come to define India's states. There had been years of debate during Partition about how best to draw new state boundaries that would turn the old kingdoms and provinces of colonial India into manageable, coherent administrative units for a modern nation. Nehru, and many others in the Congress Party, were initially opposed to dividing states according to language. They feared that language would serve as "not only a binding force but also a separating one," and the matter was shelved for years after independence. But popular will built steadily in favor of linguistically coherent states—so that people who spoke Gujarati or Malayalam or Oriya or other languages would have their own distinct states and the political power that came with them. The pressure reached its apogee in 1952, with the death by fasting of Potti Sriramulu, an activist devoted to the cause of statehood for Telugu speakers. Nehru conceded, and by late 1955, the States Reorganization Commission made its official recommendations. Gujarati became the language of Gujarat. Oriya the language of Orissa. Telugu had Andhra Pradesh, and much of what had been the two ancient kingdoms of Travancore and Cochin, where Malayalam dominated, became Kerala.

Nehru's fears were misplaced. The redrawn boundaries seemed to strengthen India's sense of itself as a nation rather than undermine it. The new states chose new capitals and built statehouses. They devoted money to the cultivation of their own languages, and young people growing up during that time had a renewed sense of what belonged to them. Elizabeth, the schoolteacher's daughter, recalled that the only time she had left her village before coming to Mokama was for a trip to Trivandrum, the new state capital of Kerala, where one of her uncles was studying. It was a journey of several hours by train, but her mother and grandparents took her and one of her brothers to the new state capital. And it was there, too, that they happened to visit an army hospital, where she saw for the first time a nurse in a crisp white uniform. By the late 1950s it was no longer unusual for people from Kerala and other states in the south to move to the north to study or work; they embraced a new and larger vision of their nation, with the grounding of language to define themselves and remind them of home.

The English-only rule proved impossible for the young nurses to follow. They relied on one another and their friendships, and they resented the intrusion of the hospital rules into their private spaces. They were not novices, committed to a life of austerity and noble suffering. They did not aspire to make vows of chastity, poverty, and obedience, and they had not agreed to observe periods of sacred silence. And yet the sisters monitored every sound they made; they listened in the hallways, in the hospital wards, even on the terrace where they would hang up their clothes to dry and sit and talk while polishing their shoes. If they caught the girls talking Malayalam, they would punish them by telling them to work the next day without their nursing cap, a small humiliation, stripping them of their status as a nurse. Or they would tell them to report to work wearing their sari instead of the precious nurse's uniform custom made by the tailor.

And yet no punishment seemed sufficient to stop their linguistic rebellion. Leela was discovered one day chatting away in Malayalam in the dormitory. The sisters decided to make an example of her; they punished her by taking away her time. She was already scheduled to take her first-year exams, but Florence Joseph told her she would have to wait and take the exam with the next batch of girls six months later. Leela was furious. By this point there were enough nursing students in Bihar to form a student association, and Leela was its secretary. The test would be administered by Patna Medical College Hospital, and she decided to appeal the suspension. She told the sisters, "I will fight."

Forcing a young nurse to wait six months was the worst possible punishment, because they were all so impatient to finish and go out into the world. They had not entered the order for life; once the initial shock of the first few months wore off, they began to see that there would eventually be an end to their time at Mokama, a future and a new kind of life waiting for them after they finished their training. The road to get there was six years long. Rose and many of the others knew little about the course of study when they arrived, other than the crucial detail that the Nazareth Hospital nursing school did not charge any fees to the student nurses. This was possible, she realized, only because it was a work-study hospital, in which the nurses would have to pay for their education in labor.

For the first two years, the student nurses would work four-hour shifts, under the supervision of their seniors, and then sit in class for four hours. They started with the menial work and then moved to the wards. Those who worked the morning shift at 7:00 a.m. would have class in the afternoon. After a few weeks, they would change the shifts—class in the morning, then work from 3:00 to 7:00. For those first two years, their work in the hospital was unpaid, because the sisters considered it to be part of their education. In the second two years, they would start to get a small stipend and continue to attend more advanced classes. But while the government hospitals paid fifty or sixty rupees a month, Rose eventually discovered, the stipend at Mokama was less than five rupees. Finally, the nurses would have to do one or two years of "bond" once their training was finished. Their stipend during the bond years was a little larger, but it was not close to what a trained nurse might earn in Delhi or Bombay. The hospital demanded two years of work to complete the repayment of the training they had received. Still, it was a significant milestone for the nurses at Mokama; when they began their bond, they became "staff nurses" and received the black bands on their caps in a special cere-mony. As staff nurses, they worked the same shifts as they had when they were students, but they no longer had to go to classes in between. They were able to rest and perhaps think about what came next.

Sometimes, when she thought about it, Rose realized how truly isolated they were. Where were the glamorous women in starched caps and stylish hairdos? There were none in Mokama, only a hand-ful of homesick girls just like her. There was no way for them to call their families; long distance calls had to be booked in advance. They could write letters, of course, but the mail could take weeks to reach Kerala and sometimes went missing. The sisters often sent telegrams for urgent news to Patna or to the United States, but Rose's parents were certainly not in the habit of walking from their village to the telegraph office in Palai to check for messages. If anything ever hap-pened to one of the young nurses, their families might not hear about it for days.

Not every young woman who came to Mokama left as a nurse. There were a few who couldn't endure the cold and the rules and the hard work, and went home to face the anger and embarrassment surely waiting for them in Kerala. There was Aleykutty, a student nurse who disappeared one day during supper. She had only been there a couple of months and simply walked away, leaving all her be-longings behind. There was the girl who scandalized the sisters when she seemed to have become a little too friendly with one of the pa-tients in the hospital. She insisted she hadn't done anything wrong, but was sent home in disgrace just the same.

Then there was the girl who collapsed five days after the August evening on which she received her cap and uniform. She fell into a coma, possibly from viral hepatitis, never regained consciousness, and died the next day. The sisters tried to call her parents in Kerala, and then her brother, who was stationed with the Indian Air Force in Bangalore, but they couldn't get through. They sent telegrams, then letters. They waited as long as they could for an answer—leaving the body in the air-conditioned operating room for an extra day, hoping someone might be able to come from Kerala. No one ever did, and she was buried right there at Nazareth Hospital cemetery. The nurses, the doctors, all the sisters, and even the servants gathered to bury her, praying over the casket as they lowered it into the earth at Mokama.

But those who survived and made it through to their bond years could finally start to plan for a life somewhere else.

Leela, in the end, won her appeal, so Florence Joseph allowed her to take her exams on schedule and instead docked her days off as punishment. When Leela finished her bond, she never went back to her life in Kerala. She and a few others found jobs together at a hospital in Delhi. The city and the hospital wards were many times bigger than Mokama, but Leela grudgingly admitted that Nazareth had prepared her well. Finally, Leela thought, this was freedom.

Rose and the others hoped one day to join her there. Rose wanted to go as soon as possible, so she could start sending money home to get her younger sisters married. Elsy was so young when she started at Mokama—only fifteen—that it took her an extra year to finish. Her training could only officially "begin" once she turned sixteen, so in the end she spent seven years at Mokama.

On their days off, the nurses would ask for permission to go to the movies in town, or send for a pony cart from Chedilal's sari shop in the bazaar, along with a clerk who would act as their chaperone and protector. The cart would take a few of the young women to the shop, where they could run their hands in the silks and the slippery new synthetic chiffons and make plans to spend their tiny stipends. Elizabeth was so proud of the first saris she bought for herself; she didn't need her father to send for the tailor to make dresses for her anymore. After two and a half years at Mokama, she went home to Kerala for the first time, adding a few extra days to a trip to Madras for a nurses' convention at the prestigious Vellore Medical College there. She packed the two saris in a small trunk and kept it locked under her bed in the shared dormitory room provided for her on campus. She woke up to find the lock broken, the saris stolen. She went home as planned, too proud to admit what had happened.

In the spaces between work and meals and chores, the nurses found time to dream and talk, and their favorite place to do that was the shrine. Florence Joseph had bought bicycles so the sisters could get to and from the shrine more easily for Masses. When the young nurses started arriving, Florence Joseph insisted that they, too, should learn to ride bicycles, coasting down the paths toward the wide green lawns of the shrine. It was the only place to go in Mokama in the evenings, so they would just walk around, past the fig trees and mango trees, and sit on the benches in front of the church and talk. This alone was a revelation: they were on their own. There was no father or mother waiting in the house, no family scandals to discuss, no gossip to spread or ignore. They had finished a full day's work, used the skills they had learned and been paid for them, and then it was done. They could be by themselves, young women in a field under the moonlight, away from their families and yet perfectly safe and content.

FIFTEEN

Miss Wiss and Dr. Kenny

The preparations for Dr. Wiss's arrival in India began more than a year before she left. The motherhouse in Kentucky, along with the Wiss family in Ohio, who now had a new mission, started sending boxes of surgical supplies in anticipation. Months before she landed in India, twenty-three boxes of cargo had arrived ahead of her, and she brought so much with her that the extra shipping costs and inland freight charges amounted to more than six hundred dollars.

Florence Joseph, who by then had taken over as head of the hospital, had to find one more temporary doctor who could help until Dr. Wiss got settled and had a chance to learn Hindi. The obvious choice was Dr. Meave Kenny, a widowed English physician with an eleven-year-old daughter in boarding school in England, who had been coming in regularly every two weeks to help with surgeries. She had spent years in India and other parts of the former British Empire, working mostly in mission hospitals as a gynecologist. She had a connection to the Sisters of Charity: she was a distant relative of Catherine

Spalding, the founder of the order. In March 1959, Dr. Kenny agreed to stay for a year.

The same month, Dr. Wiss boarded the SS *Steel Navigator,* a freighter bound for Bombay. She spent hours on deck, although her skin was so pale and delicate that she could get sunburned just from the glare of the bright midday sun off the water.

Dr. Wiss arrived in India on April 14, 1959, and soon afterward joined the other sisters for their annual sojourn to the hills of Darjeeling, the long journey that began with the crowded and dangerous ferry crossing, and then the transfer to the northern rail line on the other side of the river.

The return trip was completely different. Shortly before she officially began on duty at the end of June, the bridge across the Ganges had finally opened, a decade after construction had begun. Dr. Wiss started seeing patients almost immediately. Dr. Kenny supervised the training of the nurse-midwives, handled the complicated obstetrical problems, and started a fertility clinic, while Dr. D'Cruze, with "one of the nicest dispositions one could hope to encounter," took most of the pediatric and medical cases, as Dr. Wiss wrote in a letter home. "Needless to say, I am mighty glad to have both of them."

A few days after she started, Dr. D'Cruze interrupted his new colleague while she was writing a letter home to her parents. He had arranged with a friend of his to drive them over to the new Ganges bridge to see it up close, so she got up from the typewriter in midsentence and went with them to the riverbank to marvel at this feat of Indian and American engineering.

"This is really a huge bridge, over 6000 feet long with an upper level for cars and pedestrians and lower level for railroad. It was one of the chief projects in India's first five-year plan, and was finished a whole year ahead of schedule," she wrote. There was already regular rail traffic making the crossing, but the bridge was not too useful for other vehicles. The roads approaching it weren't complete, only about a mile and a half on the northern side, so it was difficult to get through the press of people, even with a jeep, after making the crossing. "There are fine sidewalks on either side of the three lane road crossing the bridge, but sidewalks are somewhat of a novelty here and all the foot traffic mingles on the road with the jeeps, cars, bullock carts, rickshas, donkeys, etc." Dr. Wiss looked around and saw more than the crowds. "The Ganges and its banks are really beautiful and we watched a most gorgeous sunset while there," she wrote. "The sunsets in the monsoon season are quite lovely, but this was much more so than most."

On July 12, 1959, a few months after she arrived and had settled into her work, Sister Mary Martha Wiss sent a letter to her family describing the previous day's activity in the operating room. "Yesterday started out with only one minor case scheduled for surgery," she wrote. "By the time the day was over we had had a Cesarian section, sewed up a lacerated eyelid, operated on a woman for suspected appendicitis who turned out to have widespread cancer, and fixed a compound fracture of the arm in a five-year-old boy. The last was quite pathetic because his mother was quite sure we would have to take his arm off and was most happy when we didn't."

She used all the cargo that had been sent ahead of her to set up a lab in Crescentia's pharmacy and to equip the operating room. "Our operating room is 19 x 20 ft in a well-lighted corner of the building," she wrote. "We have a good table, light, gas machine and anesthetist, cautery, suction and instruments, and two wonderful air conditioners."

The work was relentless. By August, she was handling forty-eight cases in a week, on some days ten or twelve cases a day. Ann Cornelius served as her anesthetist and head surgical nurse, but to handle this volume of cases, they needed the help of the student nurses, who did rotations in the OR as part of their training. Some of them, Dr. Wiss complained, were "exceptionally inefficient," and she sometimes grew frustrated with how much time it took them to scrub in for each new case. There were other minor obstacles, too, like the new operating-room light bulbs, which had blown out and would have to be replaced, and the lack of an X-ray machine. She learned to do appendectomies by flashlight and to check the progress of broken bones by touch. "This lack of x-ray is making fracture treatment something to really sweat over, but I guess broken bones got along pretty well for thousands of years without x-rays, so I should be able to manage for a while till we can get one," she wrote.

Despite these limitations, the arrival of Nazareth's long-awaited sister-surgeon transformed what the hospital was able to do. The hospital was still handling the same range of medical problems as ever—cholera, dysentery, malaria, typhoid, tetanus, leprosy, kala-azar, hepatitis, filariasis, and innumerable varieties of diarrheal diseases and viral infections, along with anemia and other illnesses caused by hookworm, malnutrition, and vitamin deficiencies. But with Dr. Wiss, they could help the people whose misfortunes were extreme even for a place like Mokama: like the eight-year-old girl, already married, who was brought to the hospital by her mother-in-law with a severely burned hand; or the soldier who had stepped in front of a train and nearly lost his foot; or the woman with a fifteen-pound dermoid cyst on her ovary, which she carried along with a healthy baby; or the boy who, during mango season, suffered head trauma after falling from a tree. Before, the hospital could do little more than send these patients to Patna, a trip of several hours that few could afford to make, or ask them to come back when they had a surgeon visiting from another hospital. With their own surgeon—along with Dr. D'Cruze to handle the general medical cases and Dr. Kenny to handle complicated obstetric cases—it seemed there was almost nothing that Nazareth Hospital couldn't handle. As a glowing profile in Ohio State magazine noted, Dr. Wiss was one of only about a hundred doctor-sisters in the world, and even fewer were surgeons. And yet here she was, in Mokama. As the Nazareth Hospital Christmas card for 1959 put it, "After all these years it is like a wonderful dream come true."

In the same way that the novices from Kerala like Bridget introduced a new kind of nun to the order, and students like Rose and her friends a different kind of nurse, Dr. Wiss, too, represented a change in what it meant to be a member of the Sisters of Charity of Nazareth.

Mary Martha felt that shock soon after arriving in India. "For myself the change is tremendous," she wrote. "I am having to learn all over what it is like to be able to attend most Community exercises, to eat three regular meals daily, as well as morning and afternoon 'tea.' . . . We rise at 4:50, have mass at 6:00, followed by breakfast. Because of our varying schedules, each makes her own adoration. We have dinner prayers at 12:00, spiritual reading at 5:45 followed by Rosary and supper, recreation at 7:30 and night prayers at 8:30." While she welcomed the company of the other sisters, her life could never be the same as theirs. A surgeon's work could not be bound by an eight-hour shift; she was on call for emergency surgeries at all times of the day and night.

And yet somehow she managed to fit in hours standing in the operating room around the demands of prayer dictated by the order, along with daily Hindi classes as she mastered the language. She did so many surgeries that her skill and speed picked up significantly; in

September 1959, Dr. Wiss described doing a "subtotal resection of the stomach"—removing the whole lower half of the stomach—in a man who had suffered for years with an ulcer that severely scarred his duodenum. "That operation usually took me 2½ to three hours at St. Joseph's and I was done in an hour and a half this time," she wrote.

In the same letter, she described one particular case that she realized "will probably either make or break my reputation around here," especially among the rich and powerful men of the town. The four-year-old son of a local merchant had fallen off the roof of his family's house early in the morning and was brought to the hospital unconscious, with signs of bleeding inside the skull that put pressure on the brain. He needed surgery, and the family wanted to take him to Patna, but the next train wouldn't come for hours. Dr. Wiss told them the boy needed help right away, so they should either find a car or allow her to do the surgery in Mokama. "After much debate they decided to let me do it." The bleeding stopped, and the boy improved but remained unconscious. "His recovery now is strictly up to Almighty God, not me, but I will get the credit or blame either way."

In addition to her work as chief surgeon at Nazareth Hospital, Dr. Wiss took on another role, painstakingly documenting her time in India in the letters that she wrote home nearly every Sunday. She typed out and sometimes wrote by hand hundreds of letters in her office or in a corner of the operating room, the room filled with the elegant sounds of her favorite operas and symphonies on her treasured phonograph—the New World Symphony, *Rose-Marie*, *La Traviata*.

Those letters became a powerful fundraising and publicity vehicle for the order, thanks to the tireless work of her father. Jack Wiss had already had a heart attack, before his daughter left for India, and needed a hip replacement soon afterward. As his health failed, he was pushed out of his work as a chemical salesman, kept on with a nominal salary of two hundred dollars a month. He kept the family afloat with a modest income from a company he had started during the war that made synthetic rubber and resins, but the center of the family's life was Dr. Wiss's adventure in India.

Jack Wiss lived for her letters, having watched her sacrifice so many years to become a surgeon. He thrilled to her stories of complex surgeries performed under harsh conditions. He would take each letter and retype it in his den in the family's basement, omitting some of the more personal material about the Wiss family's comings and goings, and then reproduce them by mimeograph and send them to a mailing list of people in the United States that grew into the hundreds—friends, family, a lifetime of contacts, along with all the supporters of the order who asked to be added to the list. All of the Wiss siblings were accomplished in their own way—Johnny, the only son, had graduated from West Point—but it was clear who was the star of the family.

Many of Mary Martha's letters seemed to be written with her reading public in mind. "For the information of the readers of this epistle . . . I thought you would like to know more about the Sisters I mention," she wrote, and then described each of the other sisters in turn. In another early letter, she narrated the setting of the hospital as if walking through it with a visitor: "our big white concrete building with its wide verandas," and along the inside of the L-shaped building, "a beautiful, genuine concrete sidewalk"; the dispensary where Dr. Wiss and the nurses saw the incoming patients; then the wards for the patients, open to the veranda, with the beds so close together that it is "impossible to turn around between them." The wards were divided into sections—the women's medical ward, the women's surgical ward, the nurses' station, the obstetrics ward, the tuberculosis ward, the newborn nursery, then the delivery room and operating room. "Now we are at the corner, starting down the newer wing," an area painstakingly built during the years of concrete shortages, with spaces set aside for collections, a storage closet, the smoky old kitchen with its wood and coal-fired oven, a toddler orphanage, and a play area near the veranda. "At this area off the veranda was an area for sterilizing and maintaining all the equipment, a small laboratory, another nurses' station, two children's wards, a surgical ward and tuberculosis ward for men, and our only private room."

Like her father, Mary Martha approached the world with the mind of an engineer. She brought her own set of tools with her, figured out how to set up makeshift traction for broken bones, made minor repairs to the phonograph, and at one point broke her six-inch wrench tightening a bolt on the leaky valves on the anesthesia machine's gas tanks. The hospital had a large army surplus supply of plaster of Paris, so she asked her father for advice on how to get it to set in the humid, monsoon season. She had been using a new method to treat babies born with clubfoot, pioneered by a doctor at the University of Iowa in the 1940s, which involved gently manipulating the deformed feet and applying weekly plaster casts to the legs to correct them. "It is very hard to hold them in the proper position until the plaster is set," she wrote. "They are uncooperative, to put it mildly." The results were excellent, but required months of regular visits to the hospital. "Getting their parents to persevere long enough to get them adequately treated is really a problem, even with precious only sons."

Her letters gave glimpses of India in the early 1960s, as the country's slow process of industrialization made its way to Mokama. The Bata shoe factory was still the largest company presence in the town, and she became quite friendly with the factory head and his wife, the Havrlants, who were devout Catholics and longtime supporters of the hospital. "Their home looks like something from Hollywood instead of India," she wrote. The company's officers were a cosmopolitan lot—Indian, Czech, Canadian, and British—who lived in a big compound of similarly fashionable houses. The shoe factory was later joined by the Britannia steel plant, which made railroad freight cars. "These plants have health policies for their employees which pay their hospital bills here, and are quite a help to us financially," she wrote. "They are really only beginning operations, but expect to have about 3500 employees within the next year or so." The hospital began to see not just injuries from the hazards of rural life, but industrial accidents, too. The Barauni refinery, on the other side of the Ganges river bridge, had its own infirmary, a perk for the employees of the prestigious Indian Oil Corporation. She became friendly with the refinery's doctor, and with the wife of a manager at a construction company at the refinery site, who threw parties to raise money for the hospital's new nurses' quarters.

Dr. Wiss also told the stories of the tragic cases that stayed with her, like the four-month-old baby boy who was brought to the hospital with acute amoebic dysentery, then turned out to have a ruptured appendix, which had caused an abscess and intestinal blockage. It was extremely unusual for an appendix to burst in a baby so young, and Dr. Wiss operated on him and watched him closely for days. He rallied for a while, thanks in part to one hundred milliliters of blood donated by Dr. Kenny, but "it apparently wasn't quite enough," she wrote. "I was terribly disappointed to lose him."

There were triumphs, too. The girl with the severely burned hand had her final operation after three months of going back and forth between her home and the hospital—Dr. Wiss had reconstructed her hand, and it was "about 500% better than when we started." And she was pleased to report that the little boy with the bad head injury went home within a few weeks. "He has some weakness of the right arm and leg, but was able to walk up stairs and pedal a tricycle before he left."

By October, when the annual Durga Puja festival arrived, she, Dr. Kenny, and one of the other sisters were invited by a local man, a friend of the hospital, to ride on a pony cart to view the last day of the weeklong celebration of the goddess Durga. "Of course we eagerly climbed aboard." They saw the decorations in each tola, or neighborhood, the elaborately decorated shrines, dances, games, and carnival spirit. They watched a ceremonial sword dance and a trained elephant carrying a dozen small children on its back. The highlight came when their host brought them to his own tola, "where we have many friends, including my little patient who had the head injury. (He is now walking unaided, by the way, and his co-ordination improving wonderfully.)" She knew that the sight of three white women in the crowd was a spectacle as amusing as anything else in Mokama. "I think we were as much a part of the show as the dances and elephants."

Her reputation in Mokama, as she suspected, had been secured. She saw ex-patients everywhere in the crowd, who greeted her warmly. "Mostly cries of 'Memsahib doctor, see how fine my baby is!' and 'There is my lady doctor.' very proudly stated, so I think no harm was done."

There was a private part of Mary Martha, too, that took root and flowered in her friendship with Dr. Kenny. They worked together constantly, particularly on complicated deliveries. Dr. Kenny was herself an accomplished gynecological surgeon. "Dr. Kenny can do as pretty a Cesarian section as I have ever seen in something like twelve minutes from start to finish."

After a September evening during which Dr. Kenny joined the sisters in the parlor to listen to a concert on the phonograph, Mary Martha wrote home while *Operetta Favorites* played in the background that she had "learned a little more about Dr. Kenny recently," who impressed her as an "extremely interesting and broadly educated person." Dr. Kenny's father was an Irish archaeologist with anti-imperialist sympathies, an "odd sort of character who flitted around the world in and out of the French, Irish and British armies doing archeology [*sic*] between times." She accompanied him on his expeditions, and was "educated by private tutors, mostly assorted missionaries, while he was working on Angkor Wat in Cambodia." After a stint in Spain studying theology and philosophy, Meave Kenny entered the University of London at age seventeen to study medicine, but she left for India after her internship. As Agnes McLaren and others had found years earlier, "good positions in Ob-gyn training were only open to men in England at that time," but in India "there was plenty of experience to be gained." Dr. Wiss continued, "I don't know the rest of her story since I rarely get her to talk much, but she is quite cosmopolitan in outlook, the soul of kindness and generosity, and a real expert in her work. I hope she stays with us a good while."

The pair became fast friends and seemed to share a mordant humor about their work in Mokama. In place of a birthday card to her mother, Dr. Wiss sent an aerogramme festooned with cartoons drawn by Dr. Kenny of life in Mokama—the railway station, the stray dogs, rows of patients in the wards, and a slightly gruesome cartoon of the two of them—"Wiss + Kenny in O.R."—with blood dripping from an exaggerated surgical saw. She embraced the somewhat absurd aspects of what they were doing, like their work as "gentlemen's plumber." For the thirty thousand people of Mokama, Dr. Kenny and Dr. Wiss may have been the only people who would help men with sexual dysfunction without passing judgment or gossip.

Dr. Kenny, who called the doctor "Miss Wiss," seemed to have a knack for turning everyday life in Mokama into an adventure. When the servants at the compound found and killed two cobras in Dr. D'Cruze's garden, "Dr. Kenny promptly took them and hopped in a ricksha and went out to the Bata shoe company to get our friends there to preserve the skins," Dr. Wiss wrote. "I may have a cobra skin to send someone. Any takers?" They picked up elaborate swear words in Hindi in the bazaar, including one that "described the swearee's grandmother as having had to adjust her garments to conceal her monkey-tail." On their days off, Mary Martha would sometimes accompany her on outings, like to pick up a birdbath Dr. Kenny had asked the local potter to make for her garden. She admired Dr. Kenny's skill in training midwives and wanted to record her lectures on midwifery to compile in a book, and they spent one frustrating afternoon together trying to get the tape recorder to work.

Dr. Kenny had a love for animals that Dr. Wiss indulged; she added some goldfish and a pair of parakeets to a menagerie in Dr. Kenny's quarters that included, at various points, two white rats, William and Mary, kept as pets; an imperious mouser named Raj Kumari, who kept the rats and lizards at bay in the rest of the hospital compound; four white rabbits; a pair of pure white pigeons; "a rather vicious green parrot, and the Siamese cat who doesn't quite know what to make of all the competition." When Dr. Kenny's rhesus monkey, Abe, cut his leg on a nail, Dr. Wiss sutured him up, with the help of "a few whiffs of ethyl chloride."

Once her daughter, Patsy, arrived, living in Mokama for a few months before going to another boarding school in Darjeeling, Dr. Kenny borrowed a couple of horses so Patsy could ride. She, too, would sometimes join the doctors for an afternoon "spree," going fishing in the pond near the shrine. Patsy's love of animals extended to the stray dogs that roamed Mokama, and she adopted two of them, which Dr. Kenny mischievously named Flossie and Joey in honor of Florence Joseph.

By February 1960, the two were close enough friends that Dr. Kenny wrote directly to the Wiss family in response to the "charming" notes she had received from them. "You certainly know how to produce the tops in daughters," she wrote, and hoped she might do as well with Patsy. She wanted the Wiss family to know about the "hardships" that Mary Martha downplayed in her letters—the hours spent trying to get families' consent for operations, the frustrations with the nurses in training, the boredom alternating with extreme overwork, her periodic illnesses that "worried us all last year." But "Miss Wiss" took it all in stride. "She takes the disappointments, the frustrations, the wickedness and the idiocies of our life out here serenely and sweetly and, as we say at home, 'bashes on' regardless, doing good & kind & concerned work." Eventually, Mary Martha moved her "office" to the operating room, where the two doctors could work on their correspondence in companionable silence, except for the click of the typewriter and the music from the phonograph.

Dr. Kenny's letters hinted at problems that occasionally came through in Dr. Wiss's as well. When a couple from Cleveland, the Smiths, came to visit Mokama (they were there to discreetly scout out the new steel mill on behalf of Mr. Smith's employer, Republic Steel, but had come on the pretense of a "vacation" to visit a missionary nun they knew in the area), Dr. Wiss took the opportunity to send home with them an uncensored letter. "I am sending this by them to put in a few items that might not get by the censors which all mail going out of India gets inspected by," she explained. "We have to be a little discreet [in] what we write in order to avoid unpleasantness." India had imposed strict limits on the number of missionary visas it would issue, and foreigners were under constant scrutiny by the bureaucrats who enforced India's limits on imported goods.

She wanted her family to know "that we are not particularly popular with the people of Mokameh proper, most of our patients coming from the neighboring villages," she explained. The people in the town, especially the upper-caste merchants and the assorted bonesetters and vaguely trained doctors in the bazaar, had started to resent the success of Nazareth Hospital, especially its newly famous surgeon.

Dr. Wiss also admitted that she sometimes lost her patience with the families of her patients. "Had another fight on afternoon rounds with a family who refused to let us give the baby, who has pneumonia, any injections, then had the nerve to start screaming that he had been here two whole days and wasn't well yet."

She noticed, too, that not everyone in the hospital was happy. It wasn't just the homesick young women from Kerala. They at least had one another. But Celine, who had been there from the beginning and had suffered through those earliest days, felt isolated. The nursing school seemed dominated by the young women from Kerala; Celine's only real friend was Helen Enoch, a Christian from Bettiah. Celine was now the nursing supervisor, but she found that she was not treated any better than the least experienced nurses and quarreled with Florence Joseph about it. She was the one assigned to night duty most of the time, the one who was ordered to clean up the soiled linens after deliveries. Florence Joseph also asked Celine to help the new students pass their nursing exams, but she refused. Why should she, who had done it without even a high school certificate, help these coddled young women who had so many advantages? But there was nothing Mary Martha could do to help Celine; Florence Joseph was the superior, and she set the rules about the running of the hospital.

Dr. Wiss also knew that not everyone in the order was enamored of her work. She heard that some of the sisters back in Kentucky had complained about having to listen to her long letters read aloud during community mealtime; they were bored and asked the superior to read them the abridged versions. When her father suggested that he might compile the letters into a book, she discouraged the idea. "Don't forget that not all the Community is head over heels in love with me."

The work began to take a toll on Dr. Wiss's health. She acquired many of the assorted illnesses of the area, along with a case of allergic dermatitis to the surgical gloves that she was wearing, so severe that her hands became red and raw and covered in painful blisters. She "bashed on," as ever, though, and found a solution. With the help of her father, she contacted a company in the United States that made surgical gloves made of neoprene. She tested a patch to make sure she could tolerate them, and soon had a steady supply of new gloves. Dr. Wiss reached an uneasy peace with the doctors in Mokama, too. She was elected president of the Mokama branch of the Indian Medical Association—an organization that, she explained, never met except once a year for elections, and she had run for the position of president unopposed. She posed with them in an awkward photograph to mark the occasion, seven of the doctors in suits and one seated next to her in shawl and dhoti, a cigarette dangling from his fingers.

By the end of Mary Martha's second year, Dr. Kenny announced that she planned to leave India. Her daughter, she felt, was being spoiled by living among Indian servants and needed to be among her own kind, so she had decided to settle in Australia. The Wiss family arranged for the delivery of an extravagant gift—a new suitcase. She wrote one more letter to the Wiss family, thanking them for the gift and for their daughter's friendship. She was, again, full of effusive praise, reassuring them of the importance of Mary Martha's work in India, her brilliance as a surgeon, and her kindness as a human being. But this time, she also felt compelled to send them a warning: their dear daughter was in over her head.

"Well, we've had a good year and a bit together, your moppet and I. I shall be really sorry to leave her in another three months for, stout of heart though she is, things get her down terribly sometimes." As a new surgeon, she needed the praise and support of patients and her colleagues, but she had none of that.

The patients' families resisted Dr. Wiss's advice and haggled over fees, and she had only Dr. Kenny to confide in. "She can at least blow her top to me, and many a session of profanity have we indulged in together," Dr. Kenny wrote. The sisters in the order, she explained, were fond of Dr. Wiss and loved her as their sister, but they "can have no real understanding of her struggles as a doctor. There is a very wide and impassable gulf in the world between the doctor and the nurse." She warned the Wiss family that Mokama was "the wickedest spot in Bihar," full of drug trafficking and "white slavery," not to mention armed robbery, protection rackets, violent crime, and a "terrified and corrupt" police force. "Pray for your child, for she has burdens too heavy for her young and not very strong shoulders."

Dr. Kenny, of course, knew about the mimeographs, too, and she made it clear that everything she had written was for their eyes only. "For publication, the hospital is booming, we have increased the total operations already by a third over last year and your child's skill and sweetness are a delight."

SIXTEEN

The Flood

The rains began on September 30, 1961, with showers and cloudy weather the next morning. But at about noon on Sunday, October 1, the wind and downpour began. "Rain such as they had not had during the whole monsoon and high winds with it driving the water way in on the verandahs," Lawrencetta wrote to her sisters. "It is true that in both the hospital and the novitiate building we were marooned for a week, but we are well and happy and escaped without much loss."

This violent storm—during a time when the weather was usually clear and fine, when the people of Mokama were preparing for the annual puja holidays—continued for thirty-six hours. The poor quality of the soil on the convent's property soon became apparent; it had once been an empty lot near the railway station, and it did not have enough drainage to absorb the quantities of water that suddenly inundated the land. "The newly planted rose garden in the southern end of our property was deep in water. However this was nothing to what came the next few days."

It was a rain without end. The rains far exceeded the usual boundaries of the riverbanks, and the water began to rise at the rate of about an inch every hour. "Tuesday night, when it was still rising, all cement and other movable things were moved or raised to higher quarters. There was one high spot on the middle walk in the novitiate grounds and we measured the rise and decline by this."

When the day broke on Wednesday morning, they saw that the water had reached its peak. "The sun came out bright and clear, and the water began to recede," Lawrencetta wrote. The next day it retreated further, and the next day further still. It was a week, however, before the sisters, nurses, and staff of Nazareth were able to move from one building on the grounds to the next. The water came within inches of the hospital and the novitiate veranda, Lawrencetta wrote. "We had Mass in our chapel each morning; Father de Genova rolled up his pants to his knees and waded through the water." They had enough food stored to last a few days, and it had to be brought from the hospital the same way, carried across the knee-deep water. Lawrencetta and everyone in the novitiate had to remain there, while the nurses and the rest of the staff stayed in the hospital; the priests made space for about forty families from the area in the school. They were entirely surrounded by water.

While the water rose, Lawrencetta had no news of the fate of two sisters who were traveling and, she feared, would be stranded by the flooding. Sister Ann Cornelius had gone for a retreat and was on her way back to Mokama when the rains began. She had managed to get the last train out of Calcutta and arrived the morning of October 2 in Gaya. From there she went to Patna. The two-hour trip from there to Mokama, one that the sisters made often, took more than fourteen hours, and she arrived in Mokama in the early morning of October 3. "It was still dark, there was no electricity and no coolies so she stayed in the waiting room until it was light and the coolies came." Spent by that arduous journey, she took to her bed, sending notes anytime she or the others in the convent building needed anything. "She went over to the convent after eating and was isolated for two days."

Dr. Wiss had gone to Madras for a meeting of the Catholic Hospital Association, and on October 4 she returned, wading across the grounds in water up to her knees. Her first impulse was to check on her patient, Sister James Leo, who had had her kidney removed a few weeks earlier and was still recovering from the surgery in the hospital. On that same day, Crescentia watched from the hospital veranda, still inundated with water, as the patients began to walk in for the regularly scheduled leprosy clinic. It was Wednesday, and even these floods had not deterred about three hundred people from arriving as scheduled to receive their medication. They brought the patients inside to the dispensary, because the usual place outside was impassable.

Not everyone in Mokama was so fortunate. "The flood in our part of the country was the first in the memory of anyone living," the Annals noted. "There were thousands of lives lost and property loss was incalculable." Homes began to collapse soon after the rain began its assault, and some of the people inside died as the structures fell on them. The rest carried what they could above their heads and waded to some place of greater safety.

The Times of India over the next few days assessed the damage: the floods had rolled over an area of about fifteen thousand square miles and two million people, destroying about $21 million in property and livestock. The embankments and canals meant to control the rising waters of the Ganges and the other rivers in Bihar had failed. Government officials couldn't even reach most areas, so they flew over it, to survey the loss: thousands of houses destroyed, and tens of thousands evacuated from their villages. Planes and steamer service were suspended, bridges were washed away, and parts of the Mokama railway line were badly damaged by landslides. Entire towns, like Bihar Sharif, were cut off, and helicopters began dropping supplies to marooned villages.

No one knew exactly how many people had died, perhaps a thousand or more. *The Times of India* reported that thirteen people from a family of cobblers had drowned in a flooded rivulet; at one school, one hundred children had tried to take shelter on the roof and drowned all together. In some areas, people had to live out in the open in waterlogged fields among the corpses and livestock carcasses. In the Tarapur-Kharagpur area, squads of young men hunted and killed about five thousand snakes that had been driven out of their holes by the floodwaters.

It was the moment that the reality of living in an area shouldered by the taal lands became inescapable for the sisters. These lowlands extend for about twelve miles along the southern border of the Ganges between Mokama and the neighboring village of Barh. The taal land is different from diara land, which is sandy and sits at a slightly higher elevation, right at the river's edge. During the rainy season, the water naturally collects on the taal land and remains there. When the water recedes, it leaves behind decomposing natural matter from the river as it jumps its banks, creating a black soil so rich that it doesn't need additional fertilizing. The annual flooding, in this process, nourishes land that would otherwise be unusable. It yields only one crop a year, but that harvest is extremely abundant. It's a strange sort of bounty. Although the taal lands benefit the surrounding areas, no one can live there permanently because it's so prone to flooding.

The bhumihars, the landowners who owned everything in Mokama, "owned" the taal lands, too, in the sense that they were the ones able to wield their wealth and power to extract whatever the taal lands would yield. At harvest time, they paid laborers who would come from all over—some from villages on the northern banks of the Ganges and some from the tribal forested areas to the south. Only the most unfortunate of landless laborers worked the taal land, living in temporary mud huts built on berms set into the fields. Without the possibility of permanent settlement, or any way to move freely through them, the taal lands became a place where notions like property lines did not apply. The provincial collector would never venture here, nor would the police, so the taal lands became a haven for those who wanted to slip beyond the reach of the law. But it would be incorrect to call the taal lands lawless; there were those who exerted their power over it, and a set of norms that governed everything that happened there.

At the top of this parallel hierarchy, of course, were the bhumihars, the upper-caste landowners who had once owned the land on which Nazareth Hospital was built. The bhumihars maintained their hold on the taal lands by continuously asserting their power over everyone else and cultivating a sense of mystery around themselves. The bhumihars of Mokama were said to have come generations earlier from Ghazipur, another town on the banks of the Ganges about 150 miles upstream, and they had all settled together in one tola, or neighborhood, in Mokama. There were several tolas: the bhumihars were in Shankarvad tola, and there were three others, for servants, vendors, and merchants of different kinds. These four main tolas were surrounded by villages for the agricultural laborers. Each of the villages were dominated by different castes, but they would all work on the farms on land owned by the bhumihars. On rare occasions, the bhumihars might give some land to a servant or laborer who had earned their special favor with years of sacrifice, but for the most part, the lines between each community were hard and clear.

The place of the bhumihars in Mokama is embodied in the legend of Reshma and Chuharmal, Mokama's Romeo and Juliet. There are many versions of the story across Bihar, but in the one considered canonical to the bhumihars of Mokama, the star-crossed lovers were real people, their fate a warning from the past. Reshma was said to be the daughter of the most powerful landowning family of Mokama, a girl kept carefully guarded behind the high walls of her family's haveli, the grand ancestral compound that was home to her extended family as well as to their most faithful servants and retainers. Chuharmal, in different versions of the story, takes different forms. He was her lover, or the object of her unrequited passion who refused to cross the boundaries of propriety, or a scoundrel who had stolen her heart.

But in every version, he came from the lower-caste Dusadh community, who lived in large numbers in the villages around Mokama. For them, Chuharmal was a hero and an antihero. Every year in the month of Chaitya, in the spring, Mokama held a fair in honor of Chuharmal, to celebrate his strength and virtue and to delight in the story of him upending the established order and proving his worth despite the circumstances of his birth. Like the bhumihars, the Dusadh community considered the legend a real event from the past. The bhumihars tolerated the annual festival as a necessary release—like the mischief-making of Mardi Gras or Halloween—but they recognized its threat to their dominance. They dismissed it as a fantasy for the lower castes, but they also strictly controlled how the story could be told. There was a belief that whoever sang the song of Reshma-Chuharmal would become irresistible to any woman who heard it, so the bhumihars would not allow it to be performed in the tolas of Mokama.

The most prominent of all the bhumihars of Mokama was the

family of Venkatesh Narayan Singh. Before the expansion of the Eastern Railway in the 1930s, there seemed to be nothing in the town but
this family and their property. They owned almost everything—three
hundred thousand hectares at one time—and even after India passed
land-reform measures and they were forced to divide much of their
holdings, they managed to keep most of it under the control of the
family. They owned agricultural land, but also markets, shops, and
Mokama's one cinema hall. (Years later, they refused to allow a popular film based on the Reshma-Chuharmal story to be shown there.
What self-respecting bhumihar would allow himself to be insulted in
his own property?) The Jesuit priests used to bring the boys at the
school over to the cinema when there was a children's movie showing
and ask if they could arrange a special showing for the boys for free.
The family usually obliged; it was a way for them to maintain their
status as benefactors of Mokama. They considered the sisters as part
of the elite of the town, like the erudite Jesuits and the wealthy manag-
ers of the Bata shoe factory. So they liked to believe the sisters would
not go too far in upsetting the established social order.

Venkatesh Narayan Singh's family lived in a traditional home beyond a high wall, whitewashed on the outside. Inside, the haveli was
sumptuous—elaborately carved wooden screens, stained glass, col-
orfully painted walls, and heavy teak furniture filling the endless connecting rooms. He lived there with his father and mother; he was one
of four sons. The haveli had room for the four sons and their four
wives and all their children—nineteen first cousins. So there were
twenty-nine members of the family, plus about ten or twelve servants.
They had people to take care of the cattle and the horses, maids to
take care of the children, someone to take care of the elephant. There
was a practical purpose for keeping an elephant. The taal land was
hard to navigate, but an elephant could move through it easily. So the

family kept one, and the boys often rode it to school. (It was their elephant that the sisters called for whenever they wanted to show visitors a bit of exotic India.)

The children of the family were not supposed to associate with anyone other than their cousins and were under strict orders never to leave the property enclosed by the high walls of the haveli without a chaperone. The fear was that they might learn bad habits, perhaps, but more important, it was a way to keep the family at a mysterious remove from everyone else in the town.

Inevitably, the children chafed against some of these rules. Two of Venkatesh Narayan's nephews once took their bicycles out into the village without permission, the biggest adventure of their lives. The boys fantasized about what might be on the other side; they had only ever seen Mokama from the dizzying height of the family elephant. But they had never chosen to go somewhere on their own. They left very early in the morning and in the end saw only a few peasants, a few cows, the same fields. And yet it was liberating. The family's tenants, people who had known them for years, didn't recognize them. They could go wherever they wanted. It was a new feeling, this thrill of being able to decide which way you would turn, which path you would use to direct your wheels to cut into the pliant earth. It wasn't long before one of them, Ajay, fell off his bicycle and fractured his arm. When they got back, because he had already been injured, he was spared, but the other boy got a sound thrashing.

Eventually Ajay, too, had his comeuppance. When he was a little older, about twelve, he heard that his grandmother was about to make a rare trip outside the haveli to the cinema, to see the hit movie *Love in Tokyo*. All the women of the family stayed in purdah, hidden from view, and never ventured out in public, but for this occasion, the family made a special arrangement for a rickshaw to come to their

property with a purdah around it. The curtain came down to where
the wheels were, down below the little platform where his grandmother would carefully place her sandaled foot to step into the carriage of the rickshaw. As she waited to leave, Ajay snuck under the
curtain, tucked himself onto the platform, and pulled up his legs so
he would not be seen, and he went along with his grandmother to the
movie. Later, his grandfather offered to send him and some of his
cousins to see the movie. "Oh, yes, it's very good," he said. "How did
you know?" his grandfather asked. His ruse was revealed, and he,
too, got his thrashing.

By the time they had finished high school, the young men of the
family were finally allowed to roam Mokama by themselves, and they
did so with the assurance that their position as bhumihar was secure.
The bhumihars tolerated the hospital and knew the American women
in their white habits sweeping through Mokama, but they were also
made uneasy by it, as Dr. Wiss and Dr. Kenny hinted in their letters.
Nazareth Hospital was perhaps the only place where the hierarchies
of caste did not apply in a way that the bhumihars could control.
There were lepers at Nazareth, the most unclean outcastes of all, and
they gathered by the thousands every week. Women ran this hospital,
and they treated everyone more or less the same, although, of course,
the rich could pay for a private room or for house calls. But they could
not pay to avoid death, or to quiet the cries of a mother whose infant
was born months too soon.

During that summer of 1961, before the floods, during the height of
the monsoon, a baby boy had been brought to the hospital. Bibhuthi
was Venkatesh Narayan's nephew, Ajay's younger brother, the grandson of one of the bhumihars who had donated the land on which the

hospital sat. He had been born at the hospital prematurely, and had spent the first six months of his life in an incubator. He also had a deformity of his foot, a clubfoot. Dr. Wiss treated him as she had so many other clubfoot babies, with a series of plaster casts that would correct the shape and position of his tiny feet and legs. It was the monsoon season, and she wanted to keep the baby in the hospital— she worried that the plaster wouldn't dry completely, and the mois- ture trapped inside the cast could lead to skin infections or other complications. His family nevertheless insisted on taking him home, so she asked them to sign a letter saying that he had been released against medical advice. Sure enough, he developed pneumonia, and the family brought him back to the hospital extremely ill.

On July 26, 1961, the Annals noted, "Bibhuthi, the grandson of the honorary magistrate of Mokameh, Shriman Brijnath Babu, died here and the Child's father has initiated court proceedings against us. An uncle of the child came to the hospital to get the remains and broke up some of the property of the house and used insulting lan- guage to the Sister who had charge of the baby. Sister Florence Joseph notified the police, July 24th, the day the baby died."

This was not the usual practice in the hospital, where babies and young children unfortunately died regularly. In that year, there were fifty-five deaths, about one every week. "They are trying to prove that we neglected the child and that we refused to give the body after death, that we even took the body to the cemetery for burial."

Venkatesh Narayan was then twenty-five; he had been trained as a lawyer, like his father before him, who never practiced law but had been named an "honorary magistrate" in Mokama. He expected the law to protect his family. The hospital's land once belonged to the bhumiars and they had given it in exchange for some vague promises about a zenana hospital that would lift them above the dangers of childbirth. He had a young man's pride, and he was furious that his brother's child had died and that these American women had done nothing to stop it. He came to the hospital in a rage, shouting wildly at the nurse who had been on duty, and then raising his hand and striking her. Florence Joseph came and put a stop to it. He left with the body; the child was just six months old. Two days later, the family filed a case of manslaughter against the hospital, naming Sister Florence Joseph, Sister Mary Jude, and Dr. Wiss as the defendants. They accused the women of killing the boy and then hiding the body by burying it in the hospital cemetery—a further insult for Hindus, who believed in cremation.

Dr. Wiss, in her letters home, dismissed the lawsuit as a "nuisance," but Florence Joseph was more troubled. It dragged on, and every so often for the next several months, Florence Joseph would announce that she had to appear for yet another court date in Patna. There is no record of the case until the following year. On January 25, 1962, the Annals note, "The 'Case' was to have been convened again, but we have heard nothing concerning the outcome. Later we heard that there is no one to try the case, so it has been transferred to March 29." One of the Jesuit priests had been enlisted to work on their case, with a prominent Patna lawyer. "We do not know what we should have done without his help." It was one of the very few instances in which Florence Joseph seemed unsure of herself. She would leave, telling the others, "I'm going to court, pray for me."

It was a complicated time for Americans in India. At the highest levels of diplomacy, the two countries had never been closer. Vice President Lyndon B. Johnson visited India in 1961, and Florence Joseph proudly noted that "he was convinced of India's abiding friendship to

the United States." The American ambassador, John Kenneth Galbraith, had become a close adviser to Nehru, bolstering Nehru's visions of a modern, industrialized India with regular deputations of
American experts and the dispersal of foreign aid. Galbraith orchestrated Jackie Kennedy's spectacular tour of North Indian splendor.

But this did little to help the relationship between Americans and
Indians in a place like Mokama. The sisters at Nazareth were trying
to serve the poor while remaining in the good graces of the powerful,
who oppressed those same people. They joined professional organizations of nurses and hospitals; they tried to stay on good terms with
the police and the bureaucracy. The order even entered vegetables
from the hospital garden and white Leghorn chickens in the local
agricultural fair, winning six prizes in 1961. But no matter how carefully they trod, they could not escape the anti-American sentiment
that had become pervasive in many countries during the Cold War or
the rumors that circulated about them in the bazaar. When they had
first arrived in India, the sisters entered the vacuum left by the British.
They were different; they were American. But they would never be
welcomed. India had put strict limits on missionary visas, and during
this time of rising hostility to both China and the United States, the
hospital and its leaders would always be identified with American
power.

After many months of delays and court appearances, in April
1962, the sisters got good news about the case. The lawsuit had been
dismissed by the magistrate because the charges are "evidently false."
This was unusual, the Annals note, because it was much more typical
that a case might be dismissed for lack of evidence. "But to get it
clearly defined, is much better for the good name of the hospital."
The dismissal papers were important, in case at a later date there
might be "any question of compromise."

Decades later, Venkatesh Narayan Singh and his family recalled the incident somewhat differently. It was true, he had lost his temper in anger at the loss of the child. These American women had failed to live up to the promise that Batson had made them so many years earlier, when they indulged his crazy idea for a modern hospital, one where their wealth might spare them from tragedy. Yes, the case had been dismissed, and the family reached an understanding with the sisters, but no one ever forgot, and the bhumihars had made their presence known once again.

SEVENTEEN

Arrivals

I n the spring of 1963, Johnny Wiss, Mary Martha's older brother, wrote to her with good news: he would be able to visit her and planned to arrive in Delhi on March 17. Johnny had been an officer in the army since graduating from West Point in 1946. He had been posted in different places—at White Sands Proving Ground in New Mexico and then in California at the new Jet Propulsion Laboratory—and had visited her with his young family when she was doing her residency at St. Joseph's. His children were awestruck when their aunt took them on a visit to the morgue.

He worried about his sister. They had always been close—they were born on the same day a year apart—and like the rest of his family, he had been following her adventures in India and growing alarmed at the news of her poor health. In late January 1963, she fell ill with a mild case of hepatitis and, as a result, jaundice—two others in the hospital had it, too—and it took weeks for her to recover. She was sick enough that she was unable to work, and a doctor from the Medical Missionaries, who came to see her in February, found a concerning growth on her thyroid and told her that as soon as she recovered, she should have it removed.

Johnny's trip was the product of luck and a bit of judicious string-pulling in the army bureaucracy. He had been trying to arrange a visit for weeks, but the Indian government had suddenly stopped issuing tourist visas "as some sort of crisis is expected this month," as Mary Martha wrote to her parents on March 11, resigned to the fact that she wouldn't be able to see her brother after all. But the same day, she got the news that Johnny had found a way. He was stationed in Berlin with the army, and one of their missions was to support India in its conflict with China: the United States, Johnny recalled later, partici-pated in parachute assault missions, and it was sending high-altitude aircraft parts to India as well. Johnny had to take personal leave for the trip itself, but he arranged to hitch a ride on a C-130 transport plane from France to India. It wasn't convenient—his plane made stops in Turkey on the way out and Iran on the way back, so it took him four days to get from Berlin to Delhi—but his sister was thrilled. She was still recovering from hepatitis and trying to get back to her work, but the excitement and distraction of his visit was overwhelm-ing. "I won't be any good at all this week, I can see it now," she wrote.

Her brother's visit was a small mercy for Dr. Wiss during a period of confusion, humiliation, and frustration for India. Just months ear-lier, in October and November 1962, India and China had fought a short but vicious war over its disputed border in the high Himalayan ice. On October 28, 1962, Nehru summoned Ambassador Galbraith and said that India needed help from the West. In response, Britain and the U.S. began sending transport planes with arms and ammunition.

The war was over in a matter of weeks, but more than a thousand Indian soldiers and more than seven hundred Chinese soldiers were killed in a conflict that ended without any meaningful change in the tense relationship between the two countries. The entire region, including Bihar, spent months under the cold shadow of its powerful neighbor to the east. Some foreigners escaped the difficulties; the Havrlants, from the nearby shoe factory, took a three-month vacation in Australia. But the sisters felt a duty to stay.

On November 4, 1962, Dr. Wiss sent another uncensored letter home with visitors, describing the mobilization. "There has been a great deal of troop movement, all of which, in this section, passes through here on account of the bridge, the only rail route to the Northeast Frontier," she wrote. "If the war does move this way, we are in a somewhat vulnerable spot because of the strategic position of the bridge, so everything coming and going in this area will probably be under pretty close surveillance." The sisters accepted the possibility that their convent building might be appropriated for military use. "It is the biggest, newest and best building in these parts," Dr. Wiss wrote.

The hospital raised a thousand rupees in cash for India's National Defense Fund, donated by the nurses, sisters, servants, and laborers, as well as gold earrings, necklaces, and other jewelry from the postulants and novices. Emergency ambulance trains filled with wounded soldiers, most with serious frostbite injuries to their feet, passed through Mokama. The gravity of the war is perhaps most clearly revealed in a lecture later that month given by Dr. Wiss to a packed meeting of the Bihar chapter of the Trained Nurses Association: "Complicated Injuries Including Thermo-Nuclear Injuries Occurring During War Disaster."

When he reached Mokama, Johnny Wiss found that his sister was as she had always been—tireless and laser focused on the task at hand. A couple of days before his arrival, she had performed "two major operations," so Mr. Havrlant offered the Bata company car so she could avoid the tiring, hours-long train journey and would be able to travel in comfort to meet him in Patna. "We must have sounded like chattering magpies," Johnny wrote, because he and his sister seemed to talk endlessly for the duration of his five-day visit. She told him about the lawlessness in Mokama, about the greedy landlords and rice merchants, and about having to operate on a notorious criminal guarded by four armed men, who told her she should operate soon and had better get him well or else. She showed him the railroad bridge—the only bridge for hundreds of miles—and the new Russian oil refinery that had become a source of patients for the hospital, so many that Mary Martha had learned enough Russian to greet the wives of the Russian workers and their plump, carefully swaddled babies.

They only had a few days together, but Mary Martha arranged an elephant ride for her brother and lunch with the Havrlants and with the senior professed sisters. He met some of the young nurses working diligently in the hospital and noticed the skill of those who had been trained at Nazareth. "Of course, once they have taught a girl to be a Registered Nurse, the big-city hospitals really reach out to hire them." (The order tried to solve that problem by recruiting more sisters rather than lay nurses, who would leave as soon as they could for a better salary.) He watched his sister do the daily rounds of the hospital, checking on patients who were recovering. Johnny reported proudly that they had gotten through a recent cholera epidemic without any fatalities for children. He was impressed at the reputation that she had built so quickly for herself; patients came asking for her specifically now, so frequently that the hospital started charging "an extra fee for anyone who demands that Mary care for them." Johnny made himself useful around the hospital, too, fixing all their electrical equipment, including the suction machines and cauterizing unit.

He helped them put together a new dryer for the laundry and worked with a local mechanic to get it going.

His sister seemed the same to him as ever—a little bit older, a little bit more mature. She never complained about anything, but she still had an adenoma of the thyroid that needed to be removed, and the sisters had arranged for an American surgeon—Jackie Kennedy's personal physician during her trip to India—to operate on her in New Delhi. Her brother went with her there and then headed back to Berlin. The surgery was successful, and Mary Martha returned to Mokama in mid-April. But the other sisters could see that she was not yet ready to return to work and would need a long recuperation in Darjeeling. "She is much better but does not have much strength," Lawrencetta wrote. "We are hoping her stay in the hills during May will help to build her up."

That period, in which Mary Martha's health had finally sidelined her, was one of intense activity and change for the rest of the order, and for the mission in Mokama. By this point the two other older sisters, Charles Miriam and Crescentia, had been sent home to Kentucky because of ill health. It was a particular blow to Crescentia, who had to leave behind the years of work she had put into the leprosy clinic. "Sister Crescentia has written that Mother told her that she will not return to India. Her health has not been good," Lawrencetta wrote. "She is resigned to God's will." She would have to lead the remaining pioneer sisters, the ones who had joined them from Kentucky, and the young Indian sisters into a new chapter.

A new chapter was beginning for the Catholic Church, too. Pope Paul VI had taken his seat as head of the Church in June 1963, replacing John XXIII, who had died of stomach cancer a few months after the start of the historic Second Vatican Council. The council had opened in October 1962, the same time as the India-China war, with a series of meetings that introduced the most significant changes the Church would see in the twentieth century. It was not clear at the time what the new pope's influence on the council might be, but its direction did not change. The council would lead the Church into rigorously "looking outward and looking inward," and its overarching theme was the principle of *aggiornamento*, or "adaptation to contemporary circumstances."

More than most religious communities, the Sisters of Charity of Nazareth were prepared for these changes, and in many ways, the sisters in India were ahead of their peers in Kentucky in embracing them. The sisters in Mokama had abandoned the carefully ironed pleats of the Kentucky sunbonnet for a simple veil, something that could withstand the monsoon without wilting from the humidity and damp, years before the sisters in Kentucky did. The Annals of 1958 and 1960 noted the involvement of the bishops in Patna and Jabalpur nearby in preparing new missals in vernacular languages rather than in Latin. The change was welcomed by the sisters who had poured so much effort into learning Hindi; they could finally celebrate Mass in a language that most people in Mokama could understand. The mission was, in a sense, a testing ground for the changes that would come for the entire Church.

As the council meetings started, the sisters were among the millions of Catholics who followed each day's deliberations closely. They had no television or radio, so they kept up by reading articles in the Catholic press, especially those by Cardinal Gracias of Bombay, and the bishops of Allahabad and Jamshedpur, who "have been faithful about writing and their articles are very interesting." All of them had attended the council, and were among those who helped shift some of the power of the Church away from the Curia of Rome and into the hands of bishops in India and other parts of the world.

Gracias, in particular, had become something of a celebrity in India and a revolutionary figure—the first native-born bishop of Bombay, a supporter of the Goan independence movement, and the first Indian to be appointed cardinal. Crescentia and Florence Joseph had encountered him years earlier on a trip to Bombay for the National Marian Congress, with an outdoor Mass and other events for a crowd of thirty thousand people. "Everything was wonderfully organized," the sisters remembered, and they gave the credit to Cardinal Gracias. "Pronounced Gracious and he is as gracious as his name."

The larger purpose of the Second Vatican Council was to respond to the changes that were already transforming the Church. Church attendance was drying up in Europe and the United States, and vocations to religious life—which had swelled in the earlier part of the twentieth century—were in deep decline, especially as the options available to women who wanted to work began to stretch beyond teaching and nursing. As early as 1960, Lawrencetta learned in a letter from her sister Lucy that St. Joseph's Infirmary, where several of the women in Mokama had done their training, had recently opened a new wing, but they would not be able to use it until they had found a way to fill the shortage of nurses.

Religious orders were reexamining some of their basic principles, including the rule of hours, the structure for the passing of each hour, each day, each season, according to a fixed schedule and calendar— feast days, holy days, periods of penitence, and periods of celebration. This was part of the appeal of religious life for many, but some of the rules could seem capricious. It was only in 1960, for example, that the order gave their congregation permission to write home to their families during Lent and Advent. There were nuns who attended the council, including Sister Mary Luke, a superior of the American Sisters of Loretto, whose presence was seen as an acknowledgment that one of the big issues stifling the growth of vocations was the "traditionalism of antiquated rules and narrow-minded superiors."

There were other issues, too, that directly affected the work of the sisters in Mokama. The question of who controlled the Church's missionary activity, for example, reached right into the balance sheets of the hospital at Nazareth: the funds that the order had raised for the hospital from the German bishops' council or through USAID had first to be approved by Rome. Missionaries found themselves in a crisis in many parts of the world, including India. They were seen as agents of a foreign and hostile culture, not a universal church.

By the summer of 1963, some of the changes introduced by Vatican II, including the way in which the weekly Mass was conducted, had already been put into effect, and Ann Cornelius had a chance to see this new world up close. After sixteen years in India, she had been given permission to visit her family in California. It was an epic, around-the-world journey; she left in early May for the Holy Land and then went to Rome for a week, followed by Boston. She reached Kentucky in early June, where she received an award from a local hospital, and the Bardstown newspapers turned her into a minor celebrity. Also in Kentucky, she was reunited with her sister, and they traveled together to California in early August. Ann Cornelius left for India from Seattle on August 30.

Her return to Mokama was, in comparison, a disappointment. She had planned to stop in Japan, since she was taking the western route back to India, but had to cancel that leg of the trip and arrived at the station two days earlier than expected, so there was no one to greet her. Her sisters in Mokama, it seemed, had forgotten about her. She asked a porter to take her bags and went straight to the novitiate to rest. She sent the porter with a terse note to one of the other sisters. "Please pay this coolie, at least I thought I would be met." They all hastily ran over to welcome her home.

By early 1964, Dr. Wiss seemed to have recovered her strength. She was back at full speed in the operating room, and supervising Nazareth's two new doctors—Dr. Ala, a recent graduate of Patna Medical College, and Dr. Agostina Thomas, a sister from an order in Secunderabad who had just earned her medical degree from the prestigious Christian Medical College at Vellore. The hospital seemed to be fulfilling its potential. Dr. Wiss began weekly staff meetings for the doctors, the Havrlants donated a new tube well for an isolation unit, and the German bishops' organization, who had sent a priest to Mokama, were considering plans to fund two-thirds of an entire new hospital building.

Mary Martha continued to handle complex surgeries—like the seventy-year-old man with a volvulus, or twisting, of the lower colon, which had literally tied his insides up in a knot and distended his belly. "I grabbed up a large bore hypodermic needle and jammed it through his abdominal wall straight into the blown up colon," thus deflating his belly, so he was able to breathe. "We went ahead and unwound his tangled innards," she wrote. "He is absolutely fine now."

But her letters began to take on a new tone. Mary Martha was impatient with the people of Mokama, and increasingly frustrated by their refusal to cooperate with her or heed her advice. She was weary of those who would come to the hospital only after exhausting their luck with home remedies, trusting the village bonesetters over the hospital's X-ray machines, or trying questionable treatments from the bazaar. "One of my stock Hindi phrases has gotten to be, 'If you want magic, go to a magician. I'm just a doctor and not God.'"

The sister-surgeon had completely lost her patience with the rich and powerful. "The leading families of the Mokameh area have a national reputation for being rich, stingy and mean." She described the maddening case of a three-day-old baby born without a rectal opening—a common deformity that was easily corrected with prompt surgery. Mary Martha performed a colostomy, which saved the baby's life, but the father, a wealthy landowner, refused to pay for the further corrective surgery and the necessary two weeks in the hospital. The baby's grandmother insisted to Dr. Wiss, "But he is a Brahmin child," and should therefore be treated anyway, but the doctor insisted that the family should pay the modest fee. "The father said that charging for a major operation for nothing but a baby wasn't worth it, he didn't care to hang around for two weeks, and besides he had five other sons anyway, this one didn't really matter." He took the baby and left. She wrote, "That is the kind of character that brings out my homicidal instincts."

Lawrencetta and Florence Joseph, meanwhile, were preoccupied with preparations for a historic event. The new pope announced that he planned to attend the Eucharistic Congress in Bombay that December, hosted again by Cardinal Gracias. Lawrencetta's sisters offered to pay for her airfare to Bombay, but she demurred, instead arranging to send Florence Joseph and another recently arrived sister. "I am sure it will be a very big affair," Lawrencetta wrote. "Preparations have been in progress for over a year."

Despite Mary Martha's growing frustrations, the Annals of that summer reflected a sense of hope and camaraderie; after a High Mass in honor of the first American sister to take her perpetual vows in India, everyone gathered in the novitiate dining room on July 19, 1964, for "A FAMILY evening"—candidates, postulants, novices, and professed Indian and American sisters. There were Indian sisters who were studying in Kentucky, and American sisters who had just arrived in India. They hoped the community might remain as one regardless of passports and borders. Visitors from other orders arrived, the priest gave a particularly good sermon, the nurses performed a skit, and even the doctors participated—an American from Little Rock, Arkansas, who was there on a fellowship with Smith, Kline & French, and Dr. Ala, a Muslim who had joined the staff. "This year the spirit of cooperation among the students, staff and doctors was shown more than ever before."

A week later, Mary Martha took ill again with the flu. She remained bedridden for days and then went into retreat. By mid-August, she was well enough to attend the baptism of Dr. D'Cruze's baby boy and took pictures of the ceremony with her Polaroid.

But by then she had become convinced that her health would not sustain her in India, and she wrote to the mother superior in Kentucky for permission to leave for an extended period of rest. On August 23, she wrote to her parents with the news. "You had better sit down and hold onto your knitting before you read this as I have a big surprise for you—Permission came this past week from Mother Lucille for me to come home as soon as I can arrange it, for a 3 or 4 months rest, that seeming to be the only way I will ever get one."

It is not clear from the record how much she had told the other sisters about her troubles in Mokama, but at least one of them, Mary Jude, whom she knew well from their shared time in training at Georgetown, wrote to the Wiss family in late August, reinforcing the need for Dr. Wiss to take some time off. "She is only one person and can't kill herself taking care of so many."

Her last few weeks in Mokama were a buzz of activity, as she tried to complete all the surgeries on her schedule and handle the emergencies that came up. She performed a cholecystectomy, the removal of the gallbladder, on a nun from the Notre Dame sisters and operated on a female doctor from the Indian Oil Refinery site in Barauni just three days before she planned to leave. She couldn't do everything; one sister came to the hospital with some "undiagnosed abscesses," but Mary Martha had to send her to the hospital in Patna for help.

On September 3, 1964, Mary Martha Wiss sent what would be her last letter home from India. "I am leaving Mokameh for Calcutta on the night train on the 13th," she wrote. "I leave Calcutta at 1:45 AM on Pan American flight No. 1/115." The Havrlants hosted the sisters for her farewell picnic. Her flight would arrive at Kennedy airport in the afternoon, and she planned to spend a couple of nights there before flying to Columbus. "Don't try to come to New York to meet me," she wrote. "We can call you as soon as the flight arrangements are made, and meet me in Columbus."

She told her parents not to expect any more letters. She had too much work to finish and wasn't sure what she would say to her superiors at the convent. "I won't have any definite plans for the rest of my stay until I get to Nazareth and talk to Mother Lucille. The only thing definite so far is that I plan to attend the American College of Surgeons Convention in Chicago," she wrote. "Life is too hectic at the moment, and I am sure it won't let up until I get on that blessed plane, to which I am looking forward more every minute."

EIGHTEEN

Departures

The Air India jet from Rome to Bombay, an ordinary commercial flight, landed on December 2, 1964. Pope Paul VI stepped out onto the tarmac, pressing his palms together in namaste. He was greeted by dignitaries, including the daughter of Prime Minister Nehru, Indira Gandhi, draped in a severe black sari. Nehru had died months earlier, and she was still in mourning. More than three hundred thousand people had come together in Bombay, including some standing on the roof of the airport, to catch a glimpse of the new pope.

They gathered in an open-air cathedral for Mass, where 3,600 children made their First Communion at an outdoor service and 130 deacons from Kerala were ordained as priests. These young men were initiated into the priesthood, wearing vestments in brilliant yellows and pinks. Women in the crowd wore fashionable bouffant hairdos and sleeveless blouses as the pope made his way to the altar in an open-top car. It was only the second time any pope had traveled beyond Europe—the first was the pope's visit to the Holy Land at the beginning of that year.

The Vatican tried to emphasize that the pope was not making a state visit—that he was coming as a "pilgrim" and to attend the Thirty-Eighth International Eucharistic Congress organized by Cardinal Gracias. He told the cardinal that his model for the trip would be the "utter simplicity" of Mohandas Gandhi. He spent sixty-seven hours in India and gave separate audiences to lay nurses, brothers, sisters, priests, and bishops, in addition to the well-publicized, tearjerking visits to hospitals and orphanages and the Basilica of Our Lady on the Mount in Bandra, the Catholic enclave of Bombay. He met the poor, especially children, from all of the great city's religious communities.

The choices were shrewd. He acknowledged the Catholic Church's long history in India—the event had become a magnet for India's oldest Catholic communities, from Kerala, Goa, Mangalore, and Bombay. But he was also demonstrating a subtle alignment of the Vatican with the newly decolonized world, standing apart from the Cold War powers and their seemingly relentless march toward nuclear catastrophe. He gestured to the urgent international questions—poverty, human rights, war and conflict—that he thought would show the Church's connection to the people of Africa and Asia. "Would that the nations could cease the arms race . . . contribute even a part of [the] expenditures for arms to a great world fund for the relief of many problems of nutrition, shelter and medical care which affect so many people," he said. "Are we not all one in this struggle for a better world?"

Calling himself "the missionary pope" a few weeks before his visit to India, he made the unusual step of attending a working session of the council on Catholic missions, the only one he would attend and possibly a signal of its importance. He was trying to strike a delicate position—to assert the importance of the church in a place that had both an old tradition and missionaries who had been there for generations. In announcing the trip, he tried to redefine what it meant to be a missionary: "Yes, the Pope is becoming a missionary, which means a witness, a shepherd, an apostle on the move."

The Hindu chauvinist movement, which had grown in power since Nehru's death, opposed the entire visit as yet another attempt to convert Indians and launched a campaign to stop it. But it had little effect; the Indian prime minister, Lal Bahadur Shastri, and the vice president, Zakir Hussein, came to greet the pope at the airport as a show of support. The event was such a popular spectacle that *The Examiner Press* in Bombay sold out of their first printing of commemorative photos of the event—forty-five dollars for two hundred pictures—and had to print more.

Meanwhile, Mary Martha had arrived as planned in New York. Her youngest sister, Margaret, who was working in Washington, traveled to New York to the airport to meet her. "I was thrilled. I knew she was ill. She looked so pale, so tired," Margaret recalled years later. It was hard to see how much weight she had lost; the habit hid so much. "But she just talked and talked and talked." Mary Martha told her sister that it was wonderful to talk to someone again in English. It was always an effort to think and speak in Hindi, and this was the first time in years that Mary Martha had released herself from the mental and emotional pressure to inhabit this second language as fully as possible.

Margaret stayed with her in the airport for just a few hours. Mary Martha stayed in New York and then went on to St. Louis, to be admitted to the hospital to be treated for a form of amoebic dysentery, the infection that weakened her after so many other illnesses. She had had two hernias, two episodes of heatstroke, and chronic back pain from the long hours spent standing at and lifting patients onto the operating table, in addition to the recent bout of hepatitis.

Once recovered, Mary Martha spent some time with her parents and siblings at home in Columbus. It was the first time the Wiss siblings had been in the same spot in years, and there is one precious photograph of the four of them, with Mary in her habit, in the fall of 1964. She didn't say she was thinking of leaving—certainly not to her father—but she had to make a choice. As she knew when she accepted the mission to India, the order did not allow sisters to work as doctors unless they were missionaries. Although the Sisters of Charity had made a number of adaptations to the realities of life in India, they held to that basic principle. That was the understanding she had made with them when she accepted their years of support, through finishing her degree, through medical school and years of residency. If she went back to India, the order's only mission, to continue her calling as a doctor, she feared that she would never recover her health. But if she came back to the United States, she could no longer be a doctor. She could join the ranks of hospital administrators, whom she called useless bureaucrats, or try to make peace with life as an ordinary sister.

She went back to Kentucky but said nothing to her family or to the other sisters in India about her plans. In January, they were still optimistic that Mary Martha would return. She wrote them a letter saying that she was feeling better, although not quite well enough to return to Mokama. "A few more months should help her wonderfully," Lawrencetta wrote in a letter to her sisters.

The following month, Jack Wiss died, and something in Mary

Martha seemed to break. She went home for the funeral, and her sister remembered the scene vividly. There was a crowd of mourners in
the house for a reception, and Margaret was preoccupied. Someone
was weeping hysterically, and Margaret was tending to her. But then
someone told her that Mary Martha had fainted. She had the flu, but
of course, she didn't tell anyone. Margaret went upstairs, walked into
the room where the mourners had taken Mary Martha to rest, and
found her sitting on the bed. She turned, and Margaret was startled
to see her sister's pale hair, roughly cropped at the nape of her neck.
She had removed her veil and was calmly sipping a beer.

This was the moment that Sister Mary Martha began the process
of becoming only Dr. Wiss.

As with so many things in the order, the process of leaving it was
slow and methodical. It began with a letter written on July 2, 1965,
by the mother general of the order to the bishop of Marquette, Michigan, informing him that Sister Mary Martha Wiss would be staying
temporarily with her sister in his diocese in Newberry, Michigan.
Later that month, Mother Lucille wrote to the Vatican, to the prefect
of the Sacred Congregation for the Affairs of Religious, informing
him that Dr. Wiss was "asking for a dispensation from simple, perpetual vows." She was then thirty-nine years old.

The letter, in two short paragraphs, captured two decades of a
woman's struggle to fulfill two needs locked in a conflict she could
not resolve: "Since it was her desire, permission was asked and received that she study medicine and she graduated from Georgetown
University Medical School in 1953. She went to India in 1959 and
since that time she has been the chief surgeon in our hospital at Mokameh Junction in the Patna District. In September 1964 she asked to
return to the United States for medical and psychiatric care and until
her dismissal about a month ago, she has been under the care of

doctors, who now recommend that she seek the dispensation. We regret that this action seems necessary but we feel that it is for the best interest of both Sister and of the Congregation. The Council General, therefore, approved of the petition and asks that it be granted."

Three weeks later, a dispensation from her vows and an "indult of secularization" had made its way back to the motherhouse from Rome, passed on by the Archbishop of Louisville with a request that Mary Martha write to accept the dispensation within ten days. She wrote back almost immediately, acknowledging "the return of my dowry"— the money she had brought with her into the congregation—"a suitable wardrobe, and a gift of $300 from the congregation." That last was not required, but it was a sign of the goodwill from the order she had served so faithfully for nearly twenty years.

Margaret and Mary Martha spent the summer together in Upper Michigan. The youngest Wiss sibling, Margaret also had a degree in the sciences from Ohio State. Her office, in Washington, had sent her to do field work on a United States government geodetic survey, creating super-accurate maps, sometimes using measurements from the satellites that had just begun orbiting the earth. In Michigan, she was taking measurements for latitude and longitude readings to create benchmarks for surveyors, and the work required her to climb up high towers to take readings from the mounted instruments. She liked to go up at night, when there was less infrared interference, and Mary Martha climbed the towers with her.

They spent the summer that way, Margaret working and Mary Martha tagging along. She let her hair grow, and they explored Mackinac Island, going for long walks, cooking, hiking, seeing the parks and flowers. Margaret met a young man in the Coast Guard, her future husband, and introduced him to her sister for her approval. She hoped Mary Martha might return home to Ohio, but she was set on returning to Kentucky. She wanted to be a surgeon again, and everyone she knew in medicine was there. "If she was sad, she didn't show it," Margaret remembered. "She just seemed like herself."

Even before she had gotten her dispensation from the Vatican, Mary Martha had been looking for another way to use her skills as a surgeon in a way that felt true to her calling. She heard about a position as medical director for the Frontier Nursing Service in Leslie County, one of the poorest in Kentucky. The group was, like the Sisters of Charity, a minor legend in the state, serving rural counties with little access to health care other than the clinics run by the FNS. Their nurses reached the most remote counties on horseback, and they quickly accepted Dr. Wiss. As the director wrote to the order, "From what she writes, I would judge that she has had just the kind of experience in India which we need."

For years afterward, Margaret tried to understand why her sister left. In all those years of training, she had never said anything negative about the sisters who ran the order, except for one incident, when she was still a candidate in Kentucky, and her mother happened to comment that she didn't write home very often. The sister in charge heard about it and took Mary to task. Mary was angry, as was her mother, who never intended her to be punished. She always said that of the three vows, poverty, chastity, and obedience, the last one was the hardest. It was convenient not to have money or things, and temptations faded over time. But Mary found it hard to have her life determined by other people. For women like her, obedience was difficult.

Word moved quickly around Leslie County about the new doctor who had just arrived. Dr. Pauline Fox was the local public health officer, and a classmate urged her to take Dr. Wiss under her wing and help her adjust to life outside the Sisters of Charity. Dr. Wiss was thin, depressed, and needed help. "By the time she came back to Kentucky, she was totally wore out," Dr. Fox remembered. She took her shopping: Dr. Wiss needed new blouses, and although she gravitated toward the dark blues and browns that she had been used to in the convent, her new friend encouraged her to try bright colors and patterns. It was wonderful, Dr. Fox thought, to watch Dr. Wiss blossom. She was sad and unsure about life after the convent, but the two doctors soon became partners, in life and in work. They moved from Leslie County to Pikeville, about a hundred miles east, in coal country, and Dr. Wiss became the only surgeon in Pike County, raising orchids in the garden of the house they shared, just as her father had.

Mokama had prepared her well. Here, too, she found her share of memorable cases, Dr. Fox recalled, like the woman whose baby had been left too long pressing against her perineum during childbirth; Dr. Wiss reconstructed her pelvic floor so she and her husband could have sex again. Or the man who had killed his mother's boyfriend with a knife—the only time she had seen someone in Kentucky who knew how to use a knife the way they did in Mokama. Or the state trooper who came to Dr. Wiss carrying his niece in his arms—her face had somehow been slashed by a scythe. Dr. Wiss didn't talk often to Dr. Fox about India; she sometimes mentioned the unbearable heat and the people she met and the little toy train that went up into the hills at Darjeeling. She never spoke ill of her life with the order or expressed any bitterness about leaving.

If she had waited just a year or two, things might have been different for her. Just two months after she left the order, in October 1965, two of the last Vatican II documents were promulgated, ones that would have a profound impact on the work of the Sisters of Charity of Nazareth in Mokama. The decrees on religious life and on mis-

sionary activity were not necessarily prescriptive, but the order interpreted them to mean that the lives of their sisters would be different.
They would be more directly involved in the decisions about their
own work. The sisters, not priests or the mother general or a council
in the order, would decide how they would answer God's call. And
the daily life of the mission would no longer be so rigidly determined
by the rule of hours.

The New York Times published pages worth of translated excerpts from the decrees. "The manner of living, praying and working
should be suitably adapted everywhere, but especially in mission ter-
ritories, to the modern physical and psychological circumstances of
the members," as well as "the demands of culture and social and economic circumstances."

Religious communities that served an apostolic function, rather
than those that dedicated themselves to the contemplative life, were
called to "adjust their rules and customs to fit the demands of the apos-
tolate to which they are dedicated." Other parts of the decree loosened
the notion of "cloister" so that the strict demands on the sisters' time—
to spend hours every day in silence and prayer regardless of the demands of patients or hospital—were eased. "The religious habit, an
outward mark of consecration to God, should be simple and modest,
poor and at the same time becoming."

Missionary work, too, would change. "Now that the era of colo-
nialism and imperialism had come to an end, *aggiornamento* was
particularly urgent. Accommodation to local cultures and circumstances was essential." The documents of the council called for the
Church to reconceive of its missionary work from something directed
from Rome to a looser structure of "new" churches, with more au-
tonomy, adapting themselves more completely to local customs and
traditions.

All these changes came too late for Dr. Wiss. But she was not one to go through life with regrets. She made up her mind to leave, and she did not look back.

The order wasted no time in putting the changes of the Second Vatican Council into effect. One of the other sisters who had joined with Bridget, Sister Anne Elizabeth Elambalathottyil, had become a pharmacist under Crescentia's guidance. Now that the order could decide what training its sisters needed, in 1965 they sent Anne Elizabeth to Bangalore to study medicine. She came back six years later to serve as the hospital's gynecologist.

Mary Martha had been right to fear that Mokama would not be able to hold on to the young nurses from Kerala. Leela went with a group of about five of the earliest nursing students, who applied for jobs in the big hospitals in New Delhi. They were all accepted, and they went to the city together. "It was good," Leela remembered. "That's the freedom, when you come to Delhi." Leela and her classmates marked a path for the girls who graduated after them. They helped Elizabeth, Rose, and Elsy submit their applications by mail, and told them to look for a telegram informing them that it was time to come to Delhi for their interviews. Elizabeth briefly went back to Kerala after she graduated, but she knew she wouldn't have to wait long. Her future was waiting for her. "Once they interview you—it's sure for a job," she remembered. "I stayed home maybe three weeks, that's it."

Celine found a different path out of Mokama. Her friend Helen had heard that the infirmary for the refinery workers in Barauni, on the other side of the Ganges, was hiring nurses. The chief medical officer came to talk to Helen and decided to hired both of them as staff nurses, with recommendations from Dr. Wiss. Celine crossed the Ganges bridge to a new life as a proud employee of the Indian Oil Corporation, taking care of the other men and women who were building the new nation.

The mission at Mokama continued, energized by the changes in the Church. In April 1965, Lawrencetta made a trip to Goa for a meeting of Catholic superiors from around India. There was a new steamer service connecting Goa and Bombay, and Lawrencetta decided to give it a try. She wrote to her family from the ship as the whitecaps rolled by, and was thrilled, after nearly twenty years in the mission, to take in a view of India she had never seen before. On her journey from Kentucky to India, they had traveled southward along the coast, looking anxiously toward the land that would become their new home. This time, she went in the other direction, with the now familiar Indian coastline on one side, and on the other, an endless unknown. "On the right side we never lose sight of land, although at times, it looks like we are about a mile and a half or two miles out," Lawrencetta wrote. "On the other side, there is the vast expanse of the ocean."

On the other side of that ocean, more change was on its way. In October 1965, President Lyndon Baines Johnson helicoptered to Liberty Island to deliver a speech at the foot of the great statue. He had come to welcome a new era with a law, the Hart-Cellar Act, that would, after decades of political struggle, dismantle the racist policies that had defined who could enter America and lay claim to it. Johnson was riding the momentum of the civil rights movement, and he was motivated to make good on the Cold War promise that America was the true beacon of equality. While eliding the presence of America's Indigenous people, Johnson framed the new law as a fulfillment of the nation's first principles: "When the earliest settlers poured into a wild continent there was no one to ask them where they came from. The only question was: Were they sturdy enough to make the journey, were they strong enough to clear the land, were they enduring enough to make a home for freedom, and were they brave enough to die for liberty if it became necessary to do so?"

That message echoed around the world, and among the millions who heard it were the young nurses who had studied in Mokama. Rose, Elizabeth, and Elsy had already come so far, from their villages in Kerala to the badlands of Mokama and then to the sprawling, dust-choked metropolis of New Delhi. Why not venture farther? One by one, they found work as nurses at hospitals in New York City. They supported one another through those first difficult years, and their time in Mokama had prepared them well. They learned how to ride the subways and drive cars, speak American English, and raise children who would make their own way in the world.

Elsy's journey to America was particularly arduous. She came by herself to New York in 1974, leaving her husband and their children behind in Delhi. She took the only job she could find, in a psychiatric hospital in upstate New York, and worked night shifts there, again living in a nurses' dormitory, until she had passed her licensing exams and saved enough money to secure a visa for her family. It took six months, and her daughters were only two and three years old at the time, so she worried, in her letters home to her husband, that they would forget her. Of course they didn't forget her, and her family later joined her in New York.

When they were older, her girls would occasionally catch a glimpse of those years in Mokama. The way she pronounced certain words in Hindi with the inflection of someone from Bihar; her fondness for oatmeal made creamy and sweet with butter and milk, the way it was served at Nazareth; and her insistence on always wearing a watch with a second hand. As the sisters in Mokama liked to say, a nurse without a proper watch isn't worth much.

I am the oldest of Elsy's daughters, and I carried all this with me as I wrote this story, the story of women who were sturdy enough for the journey and everything that followed.

Conclusion

When I started working on this book in 2016, describing to friends the remarkable story of Nazareth Hospital, one of the most frequent questions I heard was, "Is the hospital still there?"

The simple answer is yes. The last time I visited Mokama, in 2018, I stayed in a guest room at the convent and walked through the Nazareth Hospital campus, where I saw many of the original buildings; the remnants of the original woodstove; the mango trees where people waited at the gate; and the closed-up well in the center of the courtyard. The contours of the town are still recognizable. I walked from the railway station through the narrow lanes between the railway workers' colony and the convent, marveled at the elaborately carved woodwork in the ancestral home of one of the powerful bhumihar families, and traveled over the Ganges bridge to the oil refinery in Barauni.

But the presence of the hospital is not as essential to the town as it once was. Thousands of people from Mokama and the surrounding villages still come to Nazareth Hospital for medical care, but by the 1990s, there were many more hospitals and private clinics in Mokama and Patna that could provide the same services. Those who could afford it often preferred to go to these private hospitals rather than mix with the poor and the extremely ill, for whom Nazareth is still the only option.

Many of the sisters I met in Mokama had, themselves, become disillusioned with the model of the big, Western hospital. The things that patients still needed most—vaccines, maternal health, reliable treatments for infectious diseases—are in many cases the same things that Nazareth Hospital has provided since its founding. So instead they have shifted their focus to village health clinics, HIV screening, and in recent years, hospice care. Parts of the hospital building have been turned over to a school and training center for girls who have had trouble with the law or with their families. There has even been talk of closing down the building altogether—it was expensive to run, and as difficult as ever to find doctors willing to work there. After an outcry from the community, the sisters decided to keep an outpatient clinic running. (Sister Anne Elizabeth, one of the first Indian sister-doctors, whom Mary Martha Wiss had helped train, had come out of retirement to see patients.) They covered the costs by turning an unused wing into a "wellness center" offering ayurvedic treatments and meditation for a fee, determined as ever to be self-sufficient.

In the spring of 2021, when the coronavirus pandemic devastated India, the small clinic at Nazareth Hospital did what it could. There was only one doctor, Sister Shanti, and she was on her own as Covid patients filled the beds. In April, she handled more than two thousand cases, working almost around the clock. The order had to counter a misinformation campaign implying that the hospital was lying idle while Mokama suffered, so they put out messages on social media, trying to assure the community that, in fact, they were doing all they could and would do even more if only they had another doctor. As they wrote in a Facebook message: "It is a very good place for couples to work for there is a good English medium school attached to the hospital. Nazareth Hospital needs trained qualified doctors and nurses to function to its full capacity."

Everything they did was guided not by attachment to the past but a sense of purpose and determination to face the future. That, much more than the buildings that occupy those acres near the railway station, are the true legacy of Nazareth Hospital. It lives in every woman who has walked through its doors. They are women who took hold of uncertainty, saw a void, and would not let go until they had shaped it into something closer to the life they desired.

Ruth Prawer Jhabvala's 1956 novel, *The Nature of Passion*, follows a family of Partition refugees in New Delhi, years after the initial trauma, after the patriarch has established himself as one of the biggest contractors in the city. He luxuriates in his wealth and the power and deference that come with it. And yet, despite all this accumulation, his mind is not at peace. "Something had always been driving him on, he did not know what."

For years, he told himself that it was his children and their comfort that motivated him, but having achieved that, he slowly realized this wasn't true. He could never imagine withdrawing quietly into retirement; Partition had cut him off from his past. He had left his home and had nowhere to go but the city in which he had finally made his home. "He had to die there because, like any outcast, he had nowhere to go back to. Retreat was impossible for him."

As I wrote about the women of Nazareth, all of them similarly thrown into the chaos of India after Partition, I asked myself the same question: What was driving them on? For the missionaries and nuns in this story, it might seem obvious: religious fervor, a desire to "save" the poor Indians they encountered in Mokama and bring them into the light of God's presence. As for the Indian women, perhaps they were, like the patriarch in Jhabvala's book, simply trying to find comfort for themselves, and later, their children.

But those answers are wholly inadequate to explain the difference between those who leave and those who stay. For all those sisters who eagerly volunteered to board a ship into the unknown, there were hundreds more who did not. For the millions who left their homes during Partition and in those early years afterward, there were hundreds of millions more who remained.

In their letters and in their own words, the women of Nazareth were clear, although not always explicit, about what motivated them. It was ambition and longing, passion and hunger. Not for what they would find in Mokama—they knew so little about the world they would enter—but for something more than what they had. These words are not often used to describe women in religious communities in midcentury America, or teenagers growing up on rubber plantations in southern India, but they are the only ones equal to this story. It was this desire, more than economic exigency or religious fervor, that brought them to Mokama, and it was desire that allowed them to endure and thrive in a harsh and unforgiving place.

In remaking themselves, the women of Nazareth remade the places to which they had come. By 1965, when this book ends, Mokama had been forever changed by the presence of Nazareth Hospital and the women who built it. They started with an empty godown, filled it with medicine and equipment and skill, and animated it with the belief that every person who crossed its threshold was entitled to an equal dignity. This alone was a radical idea in a place where the bodies of Indian men, women, and children had been quite literally starved in the service of empire.

The hospital was not simply a place where Americans gave and Indians received. The Americans at Nazareth Hospital approached everything they did with a radical openness, a willingness to allow themselves to be changed by India and by every human being they encountered, especially the young women who joined them as nurses and sisters. Their presence forced them to confront, even before the historic changes of Vatican II, some profound questions about what they were doing and why. Why had they come to India? What could they really do for the people of Mokama, and how would they do it? They realized that Nazareth Hospital would have to become something else—not a missionary hospital, but a place run by and for Indians, an institution that would endure on its own terms, and be enriched, like the taal lands, by whatever floods might inundate it.

Once unleashed, this force did not remain in Mokama. The young women from Kerala, the bewildered girls who stepped off trains in the dark at Mokama Junction, found in that crucible everything they needed to become themselves—an identity separate from their families, necessary skills, and a circle of friends who would sustain them for the rest of their lives. When they received their nursing certificates and had paid off their bonds, most of them left Mokama for nursing jobs in India's big cities, in Bombay and Delhi. They became part of another great exodus in the 1960s and '70s, of people moving from one part of India to another, leaving behind the life that fate had assigned to them and choosing one for themselves.

It was a tender time for this young country; the ruptures of Partition were less than a generation old. But if Partition had cleaved India in two, this wave of people moved back and forth between village and city the way a weaver moves his shuttle through the weft of a fabric. It would never be enough to heal the wounds of Partition, but it helped to bind India together so it could continue. The women of

Nazareth kept moving. When a door to America opened, they walked through it, into yet another unknown. But they were ready. If they could survive Mokama, New York and Chicago could hardly be much worse.

Once you have left your home behind, where do you belong? When I think about how to answer that question, I reach back to the hours I spent talking to Ann Roberta Powers. She was in her eighties, but still active and engaged with the life of the convent in Gaya. She had recently made an extended visit back home to Cloverport, to see all her nieces and nephews and surviving siblings, but when that time had passed, she was eager to return to India. She didn't want to stay too long for fear that she might miss the chance to lay down her head for the last time in India. Lawrencetta had done the same at the end of her life, making a last trip to Louisville and then returning to Mokama to be buried in the cemetery near the shrine.

They were among those fortunate older people who managed to live past the point of nostalgia, to see their lives for what they are. I feel grateful that my parents, too, have reached that station. There was a time, years ago, when they talked about returning to Kerala, building a home there on some plot of land purchased with their good fortune. But over the years, that vague dream has faded. They, too, have made their plans to spend the last years of their lives in America, the land into which they have poured their labor and their ambition. They take comfort in the knowledge that one day, it will also hold their bodies. They have cast out their old selves; retreat is impossible.

Epilogue

Sister Lawrencetta Veeneman, the leader of the six pioneering sisters, remained in India for the rest of her life. After ten years as mistress of novices and in various other positions, she retired and was cared for at the end of her life by some of the Indian sisters whom she trained. She died at the age of eighty-eight and is buried at the convent in Mokama.

Sister Ann Roberta Powers, the youngest of the pioneers, also spent the rest of her life in the India mission, using her skills in Hindi first at the school in Gaya and then throughout the mission in Bihar, as it expanded to Ranchi and Patna. She retired in Gaya, where she sat for an extensive interview with me in 2011, and died in Mokama in 2015 at the age of ninety. She is buried in Mokama.

Father Marion Batson visited Mokama often in its first years, when he worked from Patna, but was never assigned again to the Mokama Jesuit mission after the hospital opened. Eventually, he left Bihar for an assignment as a teacher at a Jesuit school in Rajasthan, but according to the accounts of the sisters who knew him, he never got over his disappointment at being sent away from Mokama. He went to the United States, where he was treated for alcoholism, and died in Chicago in 1960, shortly before he was due to return to India.

Sister Florence Joseph, who had been visiting the United States, attended his funeral.

Dan Rice and Jim Cox, the two young Jesuits who recommended the Sisters of Charity to the Patna archdiocese, served long careers in India. Dan Rice became close to the Santhal tribals of Bihar and Jharkhand; Jim Cox wrote a history of the Patna Jesuits. Dolores Greenwell, the young sister who expressed her desire to serve in an overseas mission, who was then in India, attended Dan Rice's funeral.

Leslie Martin, the wealthy, devout British benefactor who made Batson's dreams for the hospital possible, died in 1965, as he was preparing to go to Mass. He was living in Calcutta, without any friends or family nearby, so he was buried in that city. When his will was read, he made clear that he had wished to be buried in the cenotaph at the shrine in Mokama. To fulfill that wish, his nephew came from England, while arrangements were made to exhume the body. It was removed from the Calcutta cemetery, placed in a metal casket and then in a wooden one, and brought to Mokama, to be buried in a solemn Mass led by the bishop of Patna, with an honor guard of the sisters, nurses, and people of the parish.

Dr. Eric Lazaro and Babs Gillard Lazaro had three children while Dr. Lazaro finished his surgical training at Georgetown. In 1957, he went back to India for five years with his family with the help of a Rockefeller grant, to work at a hospital in New Delhi. They returned to the United States in 1962, settling in Jersey City, New Jersey, and Dr. Lazaro joined the University of Medicine and Dentistry of New Jersey in Newark as a professor of surgery. Babs raised their children and for many years was a receptionist at St. Peter Hall Jesuit residence of St. Peter's College.

Sister Charles Miriam Holt reverted to her given name, Mary Holt, in 1968. Her mission in India was cut short in 1961 by ill health.

Lawrencetta accompanied her to the United States for treatment, and after her recovery she spent the next decade back in Massachusetts, teaching high school at several Catholic schools near her hometown. She returned to Louisville and died at Nazareth Home in 1982 at the age of seventy-seven.

Sister Crescentia Wise left India in 1962 because of ill health and returned to the United States. She died at St. Joseph's Infirmary in Louisville at age sixty-eight, less than six years after getting the news that she would not return to India. In the last years of her life, she stopped practicing as a nurse or pharmacist, and instead worked as a librarian and clerk in hospitals run by the order in Kentucky and Ohio until her death.

Sister Florence Joseph Sauer reverted to her given name, Mary Frances, in 1968. After spending seven years in charge of a new clinic in Bakhtiarpur, she spent a sabbatical year in the United States, from 1978 to 1979. During her time there, she stopped in New York City to meet some of the nurses whom she had trained in Mokama, who had by that time emigrated to the United States. I was there with my family and remember the awe in which they all held Sister Mary Frances. She died in 1996 at the age of seventy-seven, in Kentucky.

Sister Ann Cornelius Curran left India in June 1973 after struggling for years with the changes implemented by the order after the Second Vatican Council. She and her sister Nancy, whose professed name was Sister Ellen, did not agree with many of the changes, and they wrote to each other about starting a new order that would keep the traditional habit and follow a more traditional rule. At one point they hoped that Ann Cornelius could remain in India to continue her work as a nurse and begin another mission there. That proved to be too difficult for a new community, so she returned to Kentucky. On May 1, 1974, she was one of eighteen women who left the Sisters of Charity of Nazareth and transferred their vows to a new order, the Sisters of St. Joseph the Worker, in Walton, Kentucky. Sister Ellen Curran was its first leader. Ann Cornelius remained with the new order and died in 2002, at the age of eighty.

Dr. Wiss moved with Dr. Fox to Pikeville, in eastern Kentucky, where she was in private practice until her retirement in 1990. She remained in close touch with the Sisters of Charity throughout her life, and visited Mokama with Dr. Fox in 1997, for its fiftieth anniversary celebration. She died in 2014. Dr. Fox, whom she called her "beloved sister in Christ," died in 2018.

Celine Minj had a long career as a nurse for the Indian Oil Corporation in Barauni, where she and Helen Enoch worked together and remained close friends. Celine had been on her own for so long, she never expected that she would ever be married. But she did and had one child, a daughter, in 1981. When I met her in 2018, she had retired comfortably on her pension from the Indian Oil Corporation and was living with her daughter, son-in-law, and granddaughter in Ranchi.

Sister Bridget Kappalumakal, one of the first class of Indian sisters, became the leader of the India province of the order in 1994 and is now retired and living in Bangalore.

Leela Thomas moved to Canada in 1969 and worked for many years as a labor and delivery nurse in Mississauga, where she gathers regularly with a group of her Mokama classmates.

Rose, Elizabeth, and Elsy, my mother, all eventually moved to the United States, settling in the suburbs of various American cities. They stay in touch with many of their classmates from Mokama.

Acknowledgments

This book could not have been written without the help of dozens of women who shared their stories about Nazareth Hospital. They include not only those named in the book but many others who spent hours in person and on the phone recalling vivid details about life in the order and the mission to India. I am especially thankful to the members of the Sisters of Charity of Nazareth who welcomed me as a guest in the convents, in Mokama and in Nazareth, Kentucky.

I am indebted to the leadership of the order, especially Sister Susan Gatz, who made the decision to open their annals and other archival material to me without any conditions, trusting me to tell their story. Diane Curtis arranged dozens of interviews and introductions, including my first interview with Ann Roberta Powers, and was a wonderful companion on my first visit to Kentucky. The order's two archivists, Kathy Hertel-Baker and Kelly McDaniels, were unfailingly helpful and championed this project from the beginning. Margaret Rodericks was generous with her time. Sister Malini Manjoly arranged my visit to Mokama, and Sister Vimla was an invaluable guide there.

Thank you also to Mother Mary Christina at the Sisters of St. Joseph the Worker, who helped me understand the very private Ann

Cornelius Curran and introduced me to her sister, Therese Larkin. The leaders of the Archdiocese of Patna and the Provincial of the Patna Jesuits also gave me generous access to their archives. A special thank you to the American Jesuit priest who spent a decade of his retirement curating those archives. He passed away after completing it, just before I arrived in Patna.

The families of Mary Martha Wiss and Lawrencetta Veeneman meticulously preserved the letters that Dr. Wiss and Sister Lawrencetta wrote to their families during the years they lived in India. A special thank you to Marcia Wiss and Margaret Wiss Thornton, and Mary Agnes and Bob Hanks; their patience as I spent hours scanning letters and photographs, and their hospitality and generosity, helped make this book possible.

Erica Lazaro also shared photos and memories of her parents and their poignant story. The families of all the sisters were unfailingly kind and helpful.

My agent, Howard Yoon, saw the potential in this story when it was little more than a sketch of a few sentences, and he has expertly guided me through the world of publishing at every step. My brilliant editors—Joy de Menil, Andrea Schulz, Georgia Bodnar, and Gretchen Schmid—made a home for me at Viking, and I'm forever grateful.

The research librarians and archivists I have worked with over the last few years are my heroes. Rebecca Federman and Melanie Locay at the New York Public Library welcomed me to the Allen Room and the Wertheim Study, the sanctuaries where I completed much of the research and writing of this book. Thank you to all the writers and scholars there, whose silent companionship I enjoyed for so many months. Salvatore Scibona at the Cullman Center also offered a crucial bit of encouragement along the way.

In addition to the people I interviewed in India, I am indebted to the many friends, family, and colleagues who were so gracious with their time, hospitality, and help with research, translation, and contacts: Saleena and Ajit Pudussery, Ein and Ashok Lall, Rinku Murgai and Navroz Dubash, Yamini Aiyar and Adarsh Kumar, Padmini Srikantiah and Puneet Dewan, Arkaja Singh, Faizan Ahmed, Amit Bose and Tudy Jawanda, Jeet Thayil, Rajiv Kumar, Dr. Nita Jha, Dr. Ravi Shankar Singh, and my former colleagues at *Time*, including Nilanjana Bhowmick, Zoher Abdoolcarim, Mohan Lal, and Deepak Puri. Sanjay Pandey helped with several essential interviews in Mokama and Patna. The International Women's Media Fund supported crucial weeks of research in Bihar and Jharkhand.

Ghada Scruggs and Sharmila Venkatasubban helped me check the facts in this book, and they were meticulous in sorting through the dates, names, and details. Mytheli Sreenivas at the Ohio State University and Manu Bhagavan at Hunter College reviewed the manuscript and improved it with their thoughtful comments. Any errors of fact or interpretation that might remain are, of course, my own.

Many friends and colleagues offered advice and help along the way: Nisid Hajari, Amadou Diallo, Ann Morning, Dodie McDow, Corinne Vanderborch, Yesha Naik, Barbara Gray, Naresh Fernandes, Milan Vaishnav, Amitava Kumar, Courtney Rose Brooks, Raffi Khatchadourian, Romesh Ratnesar, and Binyamin Appelbaum. Somini Sengupta talked me through this book before it was ever a book, and Damon Winter generously lent his skill as a photographer. Garance Genicot and Shub Debgupta were gracious hosts during an early reporting trip. Jim Dao, James Bennet, and Katie Kingsbury at *The New York Times* granted a much-needed book leave so I could finish the first draft.

My sisters, Elizabeth Thottam and Tracy Thottam, and my parents not only cheered me on but also took care of me and my daughters during the early stages of research. This book could not have been written without the support of Mithran Tiruchelvam, who believed in me enough to push me to make the book equal to the time and sacrifice required to write it. And finally, a special thank you to my daughters, Madhavi and Rukmini, whose love and encouragement sustain me every day.

Primary Sources

Annals of the Mokameh Mission (includes Nazareth Hospital, Nazareth Convent), 1947–1965, from the Sisters of Charity of Nazareth Archival Center

Biographical records for Ann Cornelius Curran, Charles Miriam Holt, Ann Roberta Powers, Florence Joseph Sauer, Lawrencetta Veeneman, Crescentia Wise, Mary Martha Wiss, from the Sisters of Charity of Nazareth Archival Center

Letters to the Motherhouse, 1947–1958, from the Sisters of Charity of Nazareth Archival Center

Letters of Lawrencetta Veeneman, 1947–1965, with permission of the Veeneman family

Letters of Mary Martha Wiss (Dr. Mary Wiss), 1959–1965, with permission of the Wiss family

Letters of Father Marion Batson, 1939–1947, from the Bishop's House Archives, Archdiocese of Patna

List of Interviews

Ashok Aounshuman

Dr. S. N. Arya

Dr. Samir Bose

Diane Curtis

Philip Felix

Dr. Mary Pauline Fox

Mary Agnes "Aggie" Hanks

Kathy Hertel-Baker

Larry Holt

Betty Howell

Dr. Nita Jha

Father Jose Kalapura, SJ

Ajay Kumar

Therese Larkin

Erica Lazaro

Ram Balak Mahto

Celine Minj

Mother Mary Christina Murray

Kavery Nambisan

Sister Marian Powers

Sister Rose Jean Powers

Seraphina Raphael

Dr. Dilip Sen

Anshuman Singh

Baidehi Ballabhai Prasad Singh

Venkatesh Narayan Singh

Virendra Singh

Elsamma Thottam

Margaret Wiss Thornton

Father Dismas Veeneman

Edward Veeneman

Father Jose Velankunnal

Dolores Vittitow

Marcia Wiss

John Wiss

Interviews with Members of the Sisters of Charity of Nazareth

Sister Sangeeta Ayithamattam

Sister Mary Chackalakal

Sister Gail Collins

Sister Mary Ellen Doyle

Sister Julie Driscoll

Sister Mary Assumpta Dwyer

Sister Anne Elizabeth Elambalathottyil

Sister Susan Gatz

Sister Evelyn Hurley

Sister Bridget Kappalumakal

Sister Teresa Kotturan

Sister Ancilla Kozhipat

Sister Frances Krumpelman

Sister Suchita Kullu

Sister Jayanti Lakra

Sister Malini Manjoly

Sister Nirmala Mulackal

Sister Alice Mulavelipuram

Sister Margaret Rodericks

Sister Mary Juliana Tuti

Sister Elizabeth Emmanuel Vattakunnel

Sister Teresa Vellothara

Sister Betty Vernaccio

Sister Liz Wendeln

Sister Dorothy Mae Wilson

Notes

INTRODUCTION

xiii listening for the beating of horses' hooves: Interview with Betty Howell, March 2016.

xiv "That's my name": Interview with Ann Roberta, March 2011.

xiv Ann Roberta was only twenty-two: Biographical records from Sisters of Charity of Nazareth Archival Center.

xiv Twelve million people: Estimate from Urvashi Butalia, *The Other Side of Silence: Voices from the Partition of India* (New Delhi, India: Penguin Books India, 1998), 58–59.

xiv one little girl: Interview with Ann Roberta, March 2011; this story also appears in Annals of the Mokameh Mission, August 20, 1949.

xvi thousands of such children: Estimate from Butalia, *The Other Side of Silence*, 187–89.

xviii By the end of 1948: Estimates of numbers of refugees from Ramachandra Guha, *India After Gandhi: The History of the World's Largest Democracy* (New York: HarperCollins, 2007), 102–4.

xix More than 20 million: "Big Increase in Food Is Planned for India," *New York Times*, May 23, 1948.

xix The assembly embraced a vision: Guha, *India After Gandhi*, 126–27.

xx "the tingling atmosphere of plans and expectation": Albert Mayer quote from Guha, *India After Gandhi*, 114.

EPIGRAPH

1 "World War II hurled us": Bobbie Ann Mason, *Clear Springs* (New York: Random House, 1999), x.

ONE: THE END OF A GREAT WAR

3 The chimes from the stone chapel: Patricia Kelley, Elaine McCarron, and Rachel Willett. *Impelled by the Love of Christ: Sisters of Charity of Nazareth Kentucky, 1936–1948* (Nazareth, KY: Sisters of Charity of Nazareth, 2013), 15.

3 worn with use: Kelley, McCarron, and Willett, *Impelled by the Love of Christ*, 41.

3 "like an erupting volcano": "Peace Sends Volcano of Riotous Joy Pouring Down Fourth Street," (Louisville) *Courier-Journal*, August 15, 1945.

4 tallied the cost: "Peace Picture on Home Front Summarized," (Louisville) *Courier-Journal*, August 13, 1945.

4 Louisville was proud: Bruce Tyler, *Louisville in World War II* (Charleston, SC: Arcadia Publishing, 2005).

5 The need for nurses: Barbara Tomblin. *G.I. Nightingales: The Army Nurse Corps in World War II* (Lexington: University Press of Kentucky, 1996), 9.

6 more than four thousand: Tomblin, *G.I. Nightingales*, 1.

6 letter to Dorothy Eveslage: Kelley, McCarron, and Willett, *Impelled by the Love of Christ*, 40–41.

6 Rose Fitzgerald, a lay nurse: Kelley, McCarron, and Willett, *Impelled by the Love of Christ*, 68.

6 ninety-three-year-old Monroe Smith: Kelley, McCarron, and Willett, *Impelled by the Love of Christ*, 26, 39.

6 ran a day care center: Kelley, McCarron, and Willett, *Impelled by the Love of Christ*, 12.

7 nursing journals they read: *American Journal of Nursing* 44, no. 10 (October 1944): 994–1010.

7 Spanish-American War: Anna Blanche McGill, *The Sisters of Charity of Nazareth, Kentucky* (New York: Encyclopedia Press, 1917), 198.

7 Sister Mary Lucy Dosh: "The True Story of Sister Mary Lucy Dosh," Market House Museum, Paducah, Kentucky, quoted in Mary Ellen Doyle, *Pioneer Spirit: Cathering Spalding, Sister of Charity of Nazareth* (Lexington: University Press of Kentucky, 2006), 259.

7 Abraham Lincoln himself: Card from Abraham Lincoln in the Sisters of Charity of Nazareth Archival Center, https://quod.lib.umich.edu/cgi/t/text/text-idx ?c=lincoln;rgn=div1;view=text;idno=lincoln8;node=lincoln8:461.

8 earliest Catholics in Kentucky: Camillus Paul Maes, *The Life of Rev. Charles Nerinckx: With a Chapter on the Early Catholic Missions of Kentucky; Copious Notes on the Progress of Catholicity in the United States of America, from 1800 to 1825; an Account of the Establishment of the Society of Jesus in Missouri; and an Historical Sketch of the Sisterhood of Loretto in Kentucky, Missouri, New Mexico, Etc.* (Cincinnati, OH: R. Clarke & Company, 1880), 68.

8 Ann Sebastian Sullivan: Kelley, McCarron, and Willett, *Impelled by the Love of Christ*, 5.

9 two competing ideals of white womanhood: Helen Deiss Irvin, *Women in Kentucky* (Lexington: University Press of Kentucky, 1979), 31.

9 Mary Austin Holley: Quoted in Irvin, *Women in Kentucky*, 32.

9 The trousseau for a well-to-do: Sallie Bingham, *The Blue Box: Three Lives in Letters* (Louisville, KY: Sarabande Books, 2014), 215.

10 a sort of finishing school: Patricia Kelley, *Fifty Monsoons: Ministry of Change Through Women of India* (New York: Harmony House Publishers, 1999), 31.

10 did not ordinarily speak: Interview with Sister Gail Collins, July 2016.

11 "I can't hold you in my lap anymore": Interview with Sister Gail Collins, July 2016.

11 twenty-four schools in seven states: Kelley, McCarron, and Willett, *Impelled by the Love of Christ*, 11.

11 Greyhound Bus corporation: Kelley, McCarron, and Willett, *Impelled by the Love of Christ*, 193.

11 agreement with the Passionists: Kelley, *Fifty Monsoons*, 34.

12 Father Charles Cloud: Sister Eugenia Muething, *Nazareth Along the Banks of the Ganges, 1947–1990* (New York: Harmony House Publishers, 1997), 1.

12 patrons were the Brown family: Interview with Diane Curtis, July 2016.

12 her "stage name": Kelley, McCarron, and Willett, *Impelled by the Love of Christ*, 9.

12 modernizing the Nazareth campus: Kelley, McCarron, and Willett, *Impelled by the Love of Christ*, 28–29.

13 direction to the congregation: Kelley, McCarron, and Willett, *Impelled by the Love of Christ*, 16.

13 explaining her priorities: Kelley, McCarron, and Willett, *Impelled by the Love of Christ*, 36–37.

14 wearing the same dresses: Richard E. Holl, *Committed to Victory: The Kentucky Home Front During World War II* (Lexington: University Press of Kentucky, 2015), 59.

14 her mother spent the war years: Bobbie Ann Mason, *Clear Springs* (New York: Random House, 1999), 33.

14 veil of patriotism: Violet A. Kochendoerfer, *One Woman's World War II* (Lexington: University Press of Kentucky, 1994), 8.

15 "extraordinary birds of passage": Sallie Bingham, *Passion and Prejudice* (New York: Alfred A. Knopf, 1989), 44.

15 "Ain't fitten work": Mason, *Clear Springs*, 87.

15 "a kingdom of men": Bingham, *Passion and Prejudice*, 52–53.

16 **Sister Margaret Gertrude Murphy:** Kelley, McCarron, and Willett, *Impelled by the Love of Christ*, 32–33.

16 **She turned Foundation Day:** Kelley, McCarron, and Willett, *Impelled by the Love of Christ*, 20–21.

16 **"Presumed permission?" It was meant:** Interview with Gail Collins, July 2016.

17 **rein in the use:** Kelley, McCarron, and Willett, *Impelled by the Love of Christ*, 13–14.

17 **"a little intimate talk":** Kelley, McCarron, and Willett, *Impelled by the Love of Christ*, 14.

17 **two young Jesuits:** Muething, *Nazareth Along the Banks of the Ganges, 1947–1990*, 1.

17 **seminary in West Baden:** Kelley, McCarron, and Willett, *Impelled by the Love of Christ*, 82.

18 **bought for a dollar:** From history of West Baden Springs Hotel, https://www.frenchlick.com/aboutus/history/wbsh.

18 **chatting over Coca-Colas:** Kelley, *Fifty Monsoons*, 106.

18 **confided in Jim Cox:** Interview with Sister Dolores Greenwell by Spalding Hurst, published August 21, 2015, https://scnfamily.org/sister_dolores/.

TWO: THE MISSION AT MOKAMA JUNCTION

20 **Jesuits first came to the area:** This account comes from a handwritten history of the mission, written by Father Mathew Uzhuthal in 1998, Patna Bishop's House Archives.

20 **administration of the railways:** Mian Ridge, "Fadeout for a Culture That's Neither Indian Nor British," *New York Times*, August 14, 2010.

20 **more than five thousand square miles:** Uzhuthal, mission history, 2.

20 **change in the late 1930s:** Patna diocese archives, Uzhuthal, mission history, 1.

21 **When Marion Batson arrived:** Uzhuthal, mission history, 2.

21 **from Lincoln, Nebraska:** "India's Feeling for U.S. Told by Missionary, *Nebraska State Journal*, January 15, 1950.

21 **an old rifle range:** "Concerning Mokameh Mission," a history of the Mokama Mission written by Marion Batson, likely in 1945, 2, Patna Bishop's House Archives.

21 **worked mainly through catechists:** Uzhuthal, mission history, 2.

22 **every twenty miles:** Uzhuthal, mission history, 2.

22 **In June 1939:** Letter from Marion Batson to Bishop Sullivan, June 7, 1939.

22 **"I have read it":** Letter from Marion Batson to Bishop Sullivan, June 7, 1939.

23 **Batson rejected that notion:** Letter from Marion Batson to Bishop Sullivan, June 7, 1939.

23 this "impossible burden": Letter from Marion Batson to Bishop Sullivan, June 7, 1939.

23 a new arrangement: Letter from Bishop Sullivan and Father Loesch to Marion Batson, September 4, 1939.

24 secure the rifle range: Letter from Marion Batson to Bishop Sullivan and Father Loesch, September 26, 1939.

24 The bishop agreed to pay for land: "Concerning Mokameh Mission," 2.

24 used for "educational purposes": "Concerning Mokameh Mission," 2.

25 "pile things up neatly for the big bonfire": Letter from Marion Batson to Bishop Sullivan, September 16, 1941.

25 "The whole of India seems to be confused": Letter from Marion Batson to Father Loesch, October 31, 1941.

25 "They think we must have the secret": Letter from Marion Batson to Father Loesch, October 31, 1941.

26 "one of the best stations": Letter from Marion Batson to Father Loesch, October 31, 1941.

26 rather than ask him for the money: Letter from Marion Batson to Father Loesch, October 31, 1941.

26 "many hours of legitimate sleep": Letter from Father Loesch to Marion Batson, November 4, 1941.

27 "Nor is it according to form": Letter from Father Loesch to Marion Batson, November 4, 1941.

28 withhold "half of your alms": Letter from Father Loesch to Marion Batson, November 4, 1941.

28 "And as for defence": "The Indian Nation," January 26, 1942, quoted in K. K. Datta, *History of the Freedom Movement in Bihar* (Patna: Government of Bihar, January 1958). https://archive.org/stream/in.ernet.dli.2015.97838/2015.97838.History-Of-The-Freedom-Movement-In-Biharvol3-1942-1947_djvu.txt.

29 "an imperialist war": Vinita Damodaran, *Broken Promises: Popular Protest, Indian Nationalism, and the Congress Party in Bihar, 1935–1946* (Delhi, New York: Oxford University Press, 1992), 181.

29 Thousands of families in Bihar: Srinath Raghavan, *India's War: World War II and the Making of Modern South Asia* (New York: Basic Books, 2016), 258–59.

29 Withdrawals from savings banks: Datta, *History of the Freedom Movement in Bihar.*

29 "India has suffered": *The Searchlight*, January 14, 1942, quoted in Datta, *History of the Freedom Movement in Bihar.*

30 should be exempt from the tax: Letters from Marion Batson to the Government of India, May 6, 14, and 18, 1942.

30 invented a "Catholic Mission Authority": Letter from Marion Batson to Bishop Sullivan, May 18, 1942.

31 his two Great Danes: Letter from Marion Batson to Bishop Sullivan, November 20, 1942.

31 elaborate shrine to the Virgin Mary: Letter from Marion Batson to Bishop Sullivan, June 1, 1942.

31 "It would mean MUCH": Letter from Marion Batson to Bishop Sullivan, June 1, 1942.

31 In June 1942: Letter from Marion Batson to Bishop Sullivan, June 1, 1942.

31 he reported to the bishop: Letter from Marion Batson to Bishop Sullivan, July 29, 1942.

32 "it will be something": Letter from Marion Batson to Bishop Sullivan, July 29, 1942.

32 "a bit of swank": Letter from Marion Batson to Bishop Sullivan, July 29, 1942.

32 paraded to the mission by elephant: Letter from Marion Batson to Bishop Sullivan, July 29, 1942.

33 "Feel like flyin'": Letter from Marion Batson to Bishop Sullivan, August 4, 1942.

33 nearly 2,500 bricks: Letter from Marion Batson to Bishop Sullivan, July 29, 1942.

33 Quit India resolution in August: Ramachandra Guha, *Gandhi: The Years that Changed the World, 1914–1948* (New York: Alfred A. Knopf, 2018), 646.

33 In Mokama, the police station was overrun: Damodaran, *Broken Promises*, 257.

33 attacked by a crowd: Uzhuthal, mission history, 3.

33 church had been ransacked: Uzhuthal, mission history, 3.

34 troops came to "protect" the mission: Uzhuthal, mission history, 4.

34 his bills for rice ran into the thousands: Letter from Marion Batson to Bishop Sullivan, March 16, 1944.

35 The governor of Bihar: Newsletter to friends of the mission by Marion Batson, Patna Bishop's House Archives, April 23, 1945.

35 "The present way is not sufficient": "Concerning Mokameh Mission," 5.

THREE: A PLEA FOR HELP FROM INDIA

37 two priests came to see Mother: Accounts of this visit in Patricia Kelley, *Fifty Monsoons: Ministry of Change Through Women of India* (New York: Harmony House Publishers, 1999), 32–35; Patricia Kelley, Elaine McCarron, and Rachel Willett, *Impelled by the Love of Christ: Sisters of Charity of Nazareth Kentucky, 1936–1948* (Nazareth, KY: Sisters of Charity of Nazareth, 2013), 82–83, quoting Mother Ann Sebastian's notes from the following day.

37 warm, polite letters: Kelley, McCarron, and Willett, *Impelled by the Love of Christ*, 12.

39 *Patna Mission Letter*: Patna Bishop's House Archives.

40 March 1946 was dominated: Vinita Damodaran. *Broken Promises: Popular Protest, Indian Nationalism, and the Congress Party in Bihar, 1935–1946* (Delhi, New York: Oxford University Press, 1992), 317–18.

41 In Bihar, the dominant force: Damodaran, *Broken Promises*, 54.

42 bhumihar-dominated Bihar Congress Party: Damodaran, *Broken Promises*, 283; Ramachandra Guha, *India After Gandhi: The History of the World's Largest Democracy* (New York: HarperCollins, 2007), 45.

42 a huge transfer of land: Damodaran, *Broken Promises*, 294.

42 caste ideology of "jajmani": Damodaran, *Broken Promises*, 74–75.

43 the land grabs became worse: Damodaran, *Broken Promises*, 323.

43 shortage of 8,500 tons per day: Damodaran, *Broken Promises*, 291.

44 less than seven dollars: Using the detail found in the December 12, 1947, letter to the motherhouse (2.5 rupees was about 75 cents), by author's calculation. The value and purchasing power of a rupee would have been quite volatile during World War II, particularly as food prices spiked.

44 In May, in Patna: Damodaran, *Broken Promises*, 321.

44 considered sending out tanks: Daniel Marston, *The Indian Army and the End of the Raj: Decolonising the Subcontinent* (Cambridge: Cambridge University Press, 2014), 219.

44 nearly two million demobilized soldiers: Damodaran, *Broken Promises*, 292.

44 paid a heavy price: Marston, *The Indian Army*, 76–77.

44 sixty to seventy rupees: Damodaran, *Broken Promises*, 292.

44 shrink the Indian fighting force: Daniel Marston, *The Indian Army*, 240–42.

45 promising soldiers that they would get jobs: Srinath Raghavan, *India's War: World War II and the Making of Modern South Asia* (New York: Basic Books, 2016), 444.

45 demoted six thousand men: Marston, *The Indian Army*, 245.

45 those going home after World War II: Damodaran, *Broken Promises*, 292.

45 The decommissioned soldiers: Marston, *The Indian Army*, 245.

45 an American site just north of Calcutta: Francis Tuker, *While Memory Serves* (London: Cassell, 1950), 125.

46 "Many Indian men": Tuker, *While Memory Serves*, 125. It's worth noting that Tuker's account, while certainly a vivid description of Bihar, serves another purpose: to shift at least some of the responsibility for the disastrous violence in Bihar to the Americans.

46 a law that would abolish "zamindari": Damodaran, *Broken Promises*, 295, 323–25.

46 In Mokama, the bhumihars rose up: Damodaran, *Broken Promises*, 326.

47 the "breakdown plan": Marston, *The Indian Army*, 232.

47 Direct Action Day: Ramachandra Guha, *Gandhi: The Years that Changed the World, 1914–1948* (New York: Alfred A. Knopf, 2018), 757.

48 Hindu landowners in Noakhali: Guha, *Gandhi*, 762.

48 Tuker described some of it: Tuker, *While Memory Serves*, 163.

49 killed at Teragna Station: Damodaran, *Broken Promises*, 339–40.

50 "Bihar had been skinned": Tuker, *While Memory Serves*, 183.

50 "fourteen thousand square miles": Tuker, *While Memory Serves*, 185.

50 Indian soldiers stepped in: Tuker, *While Memory Serves*, 146.

51 "eighty thousand or so Muslims": Tuker, *While Memory Serves*, 190.

51 four hundred thousand Muslims: Damodaran, *Broken Promises*, 338.

51 Muslim League volunteers: Yasmin Khan, *The Great Partition: The Making of India and Pakistan* (New Haven, CT: Yale University Press, 2007), 73.

51 The trains were overwhelmed: Khan, *The Great Partition*, 207.

52 Jesuits were still there: Kelley, *Fifty Monsoons*, 40–41.

52 They set up a makeshift camp: Interview with Dilip Sen, January 2018.

52 it was almost impossible: Interview with Dilip Sen, January 2018.

53 Ann Sebastian formalized the agreement: Sister Eugenia Muething, *Nazareth Along the Banks of the Ganges, 1947–1990* (Harmony House Publishers, 1997), 1.

53 "And now for the atomic bomb": Muething, *Nazareth Along the Banks of the Ganges*, 1.

54 In 1832, a cholera pandemic: Mary Ellen Doyle, *Pioneer Spirit: Catherine Spalding, Sister of Charity of Nazareth* (Lexington: University Press of Kentucky, 2006), 100.

FOUR: THE MOMENT OF FREEDOM

55 was only twenty-one: Biographical records from Sisters of Charity of Nazareth Archival Center.

55 annual "ladies' retreat": Interview with Ann Roberta Powers, March 2011.

55 "your little black book": Interview with Ann Roberta Powers, March 2011.

55 letter home to her parents: Interview with Marian Powers, March 2017.

56 grown up in Cloverport: Interview with Marian Powers, March 2017.

56 Some took the ferry: Interview with Marian Powers, March 2017.

56 missionary who had been working in Fiji: Interview with Ann Roberta Powers, March 2011.

57 youngest of the group: Biographical records from Sisters of Charity of Nazareth Archival Center.

57 "You're not needed": Interview with Ann Roberta Powers, March 2011.

57 He would sit on the porch swing: Interview with Rose Jean Powers and Marian Powers, August 2017.

57 During the war, Everett Powers: Interview with Marian Powers, March 2017.

58 had read Batson's wonderful letters: Interview with Ann Roberta Powers, March 2011.

58 cotton flour sacks: "My Story," Sister Ann Roberta Powers, SCN, July 2005, Sisters of Charity of Nazareth Archival Center.

59 "Here, sister, this is what I can give": Interview with Ann Roberta Powers, March 2011.

59 walked down the wide steps: Sister Eugenia Muething, *Nazareth Along the Banks of the Ganges, 1947–1990* (Harmony House Publishers, 1997), 2.

59 Her youngest sister, Gussie: Interview with Rose Jean Powers and Marian Powers, August 2017.

60 "The world was changing": Interview with Rose Jean Powers and Marian Powers, August 2017.

60 stained, blemished dawn: This phrase is a reference to the poem "Subh e Azadi" ("Dawn of Freedom") by Faiz Ahmed Faiz, 1947.

60 Nehru implored his countrymen: From Nehru's "Tryst with Destiny" speech to India's Constituent Assembly, https://www.youtube.com/watch?v=lrEkYscgbqE.

60 the evening was jubilant: Description of this scene in Bombay from D. F. Karaka, *Betrayal in India* (London: Victor Gollancz Ltd. 1950), 35–37.

FIVE: ABOARD THE *STEEL EXECUTIVE*

63 Left unsaid was the possibility: Interview with Ann Roberta Powers, March 2011.

63 Baltimore, where their ship: Letter from the motherhouse to the community, October 5, 1947.

64 one day of leave: Interview with Margaret Thornton, May 25, 2017.

64 three weeks to visit: Annals of the Mokameh Mission, 1947 (summary).

64 Her brothers and sisters: Interview with Larry Holt, July 17, 2017.

64 teacher who was ill: Annals of the Mokameh Mission, 1947 (summary).

64 visit to the dentist: Sister Ann Roberta Powers, SCN, "My Story," July 2005, Sisters of Charity of Nazareth Archival Center.

65 one of the other sisters: Letter from Lawrencetta Veeneman to the motherhouse, October 13, 1947. The six sisters on their way to India wrote frequently to the motherhouse, during their journey and once they arrived. Where noted, the

letters to the motherhouse are signed. In some cases, the letters are written collectively and left unsigned.

65 **On the evening of October 27, 1947:** Annals of the Mokameh Mission, 1947 (summary).

65 **At midnight, she heard the cloister:** Letter from the motherhouse to the community, November 5, 1947.

65 **Between 1941 and 1945:** Report to Congress, U.S. Maritime Commission, for the period ended June 30, 1946.

65 **christened the** *Sea Lynx*: Background on the vessel from Isthmian Lines website, http://www.isthmianlines.com/ships/sm_steel_executive.htm.

65 **17,000 tons of cargo:** Letter from the motherhouse to the community, November 5, 1947.

65 **spent $3.5 million:** Letter to the motherhouse from the *Steel Executive*, dated October 29, 1947, and continued on November 8, 1947.

66 **Operation Magic Carpet:** "Army Returning 500,000 This Month," *New York Times*, November 18, 1945.

66 **the shipping news:** Letter from the motherhouse to the community, October 5, 1947.

66 **A cluster of people:** Letter from the motherhouse to the community, November 5, 1947.

66 **Olive Dennis, the first female:** National Railroad Museum biography, https://nationalrrmuseum.org/blog/olive-dennis-innovating-the-passenger-experience/.

67 **the Statue of Liberty:** Letter to the motherhouse, October 29, 1947.

67 **She said a prayer:** Letter to the motherhouse, October 29, 1947.

67 **three weeks they spent together:** Sister Ann Roberta Powers, SCN, "My Story."

68 **seventeen knots an hour:** Letter to the motherhouse, October 29, 1947.

68 **heavy rain made it:** Letter to the motherhouse, October 30, 1947.

68 **grapefruit and crisp crackers:** Letter to the motherhouse, November 1, 1947.

68 **noticed the napkin ring:** Letter to the motherhouse, October 29, 1947.

68 **chosen to go back:** Letter from the motherhouse to the community, November 5, 1947.

69 **had been lost somewhere:** Letter to the motherhouse, October 29, 1947.

69 **more than 180 pounds:** Letter from Charles Miriam Holt to the motherhouse, December 12, 1947.

69 **fifty-five steps of a steep metal ladder:** Letter to the motherhouse, November 8, 1947.

70 **One of the Jesuit brothers:** Patricia Kelley, Elaine McCarron, and Rachel Willett, *Impelled by the Love of Christ: Sisters of Charity of Nazareth Kentucky, 1936–1948* (Nazareth, KY: Sisters of Charity of Nazareth, 2013), 84.

70 little Karalyn Burton: Letter from Mother Ann Sebastian to the community, November 5, 1947.

70 threw it into the sea: Patricia Kelley, *Fifty Monsoons: Ministry of Change Through Women of India* (New York: Harmony House Publishers, 1999), 55.

71 famous Rock of Gibraltar: Letter to the motherhouse, November 6, 1947.

71 "tips the horizon": Letter to the motherhouse, November 10, 1947.

71 explore the city: Description of visit to Beirut, letter to the motherhouse, November 15, 1947.

72 the ship anchored: Letter to the motherhouse, November 15, 1947.

73 served free champagne: Reports in Australian Associated Press, December 1, 1947.

73 docked next at Cairo: Letter to the motherhouse, November 15, 1947.

73 more than ten thousand people: Aly Tewfik Shousha, "Cholera Epidemic in Egypt (1947)," *Bulletin of the World Health Organization* 1, no. 2 (1948) 353–81.

73 noticed the license plates: Letter from Charles Miriam Holt to the motherhouse, November 18, 1947.

74 *Steel Vendor* had reached that same port: Letter to the motherhouse, November 18, 1947.

74 Charles Miriam's rosary: Letter to the motherhouse, November 18, 1947.

74 wrote to Mr. Charles O. Julian: Letter to the motherhouse, November 18, 1947.

74 the ship docked in Djibouti: Letter to the motherhouse, November 30, 1947.

75 arrived in Karachi at noon: Letter to the motherhouse, November 30, 1947.

75 The wealthiest Sindhis started leaving: Urvashi Butalia, *The Other Side of Silence: Voices from the Partition of India* (New Delhi, India: Penguin Books India, 1998), 58–59.

75 200 million rupees out of Karachi: Ian Talbot and Gurharpal Singh, *The Partition of India* (New Delhi: Cambridge University Press, 2009), 121, quoted in Sifra Lentin, "Bombay, Karachi, Linked by Sea and Refuge," Gateway House, August 15, 2017, https://www.gatewayhouse.in/bombay-karachi-linked/.

76 pulled up next to a steamer: Letter to the motherhouse, November 30, 1947.

76 jumping into the water: Interview with Ann Roberta Powers, March 2011.

76 twelve million people: Estimate from Butalia, *The Other Side of Silence*, 58–59.

76 They had just gone on strike: Letter to the motherhouse, November 30, 1947.

76 a telegram arrived: Letter to the motherhouse, November 30, 1947.

77 twenty-four ships ahead of them: Letter to Jack Kennedy, RKO Pictures, from Charles Miriam Holt, December 12, 1947.

77 Charles Miriam and the other sisters went ashore: Letter from Charles Miriam Holt to the motherhouse, December 12, 1947.

77 **railway police were far outnumbered:** Francis Tuker, *While Memory Serves* (London: Cassell, 1950), 142–43.

77 **Mrs. Julian arranged:** Letter from Charles Miriam Holt to the motherhouse, December 12, 1947.

78 **walking through Bombay:** Letter from Charles Miriam Holt to the motherhouse, December 12, 1947.

78 **a small haven of Americana:** Letter from Charles Miriam Holt to the motherhouse, December 12, 1947.

78 **a nun from Ireland:** Letter from Charles Miriam Holt to the motherhouse, December 12, 1947.

78 **an urgent message:** Letter from Charles Miriam Holt to the motherhouse, December 12, 1947.

SIX: "MILLIONS ARE MOVING AND STIRRING"

81 **utterly spent by World War II:** Srinath Raghavan, *India's War: World War II and the Making of Modern South Asia* (New York: Basic Books, 2016), 336.

82 **"the mutually reinforcing problem":** Raghavan, *India's War*, 336.

82 **a problem for people, too:** Raghavan, *India's War*, 338.

83 **ignoring the countless warnings:** A thorough and devastating account of food scarcity during World War II in Madhusree Mukerjee, *Churchill's Secret War: The British Empire and the Ravaging of India During World War II* (New York: Basic Books, 2010).

83 **"We could see hundreds of men":** Raghavan, *India's War*, 351.

84 **tickets for the Calcutta Mail:** Letter from Charles Miriam Holt to the motherhouse, December 12, 1947.

84 **buy a wash basin:** Letter from Charles Miriam Holt to the motherhouse, December 12, 1947. The letter notes that it cost "two rupees 8 annas, which is about 75 cents."

84 **Charles Miriam was in awe:** Letter from Charles Miriam Holt to the motherhouse, December 12, 1947.

84 **the "refugee specials":** Yasmin Khan, *The Great Partition: The Making of India and Pakistan* (New Haven, CT: Yale University Press, 2007), 147–50.

85 **"The frequency, callousness and daring":** Khan, *The Great Partition*, 147.

85 **Eddie Rodericks, the manager:** Interview with Sister Margaret Rodericks, May 23, 2017. Eddie Rodericks was her father; she later took her vows with the Sisters of Charity of Nazareth.

86 **two reserved compartments:** Letter from Charles Miriam Holt to the motherhouse, December 12, 1947.

86 **"impregnable as dress hooks":** Letter from Charles Miriam Holt to the motherhouse, December 12, 1947.

86 **A scream in the middle of the night:** Letter from Charles Miriam Holt to the motherhouse, December 12, 1947. The account of the robbery of the sisters on the train from Bombay to Calcutta is drawn mainly from this detailed account. It is consistent with the account in author's interview with Ann Roberta Powers, March 2011.

87 **"That is he":** Letter from Charles Miriam Holt to the motherhouse, December 12, 1947.

87 **That's when she saw him:** Letter from Charles Miriam Holt to the motherhouse, December 12, 1947.

87 **They began by crouching:** Letter from Charles Miriam Holt to the motherhouse, December 12, 1947.

88 **India's railway bandits:** Letter from Charles Miriam Holt to the motherhouse, December 12, 1947.

88 **Ann Roberta's purse:** Letter from Charles Miriam Holt to the motherhouse, December 12, 1947.

88 **"Mother of God":** Letter from Charles Miriam Holt to the motherhouse, December 12, 1947.

88 **police were waiting for them:** Letter from Charles Miriam Holt to the motherhouse, December 12, 1947.

89 **a big box lunch:** Letter from Charles Miriam Holt to the motherhouse, December 12, 1947.

89 **Father Wyss came over:** Letter from Charles Miriam Holt to the motherhouse, December 12, 1947.

89 **stay in her compartment:** Letter from Charles Miriam Holt to the motherhouse, December 12, 1947.

90 **Little Sisters of the Poor:** Letter from Charles Miriam Holt to the motherhouse, December 12, 1947.

90 **arrived in Howrah Station:** Letter from Charles Miriam Holt to the motherhouse, December 12, 1947.

90 **It was Mr. Barber:** Letter from Charles Miriam Holt to the motherhouse, December 12, 1947.

91 **to arrive first:** Letter from Charles Miriam Holt to the motherhouse, December 12, 1947.

91 **confided in a letter:** Letter from Charles Miriam Holt to the motherhouse, December 12, 1947.

91 **Celine was born in 1933:** Interview with Celine Minj, January 5, 2018.

91 **contact with Belgian missionaries:** "Jesuits and India," Leonard Fernando, Oxford Handbooks online, November 2016.

92 **they did so as a clan:** "Jesuits and India," Leonard Fernando, Oxford Handbooks online; interview with Father Jose Velankunnal, January 7, 2018.

92 **India's first forest act:** "Jesuits and India," Leonard Fernando, Oxford Handbooks online.

92 **Celine's father, Lazarus Minj:** Interview with Celine Minj, January 5, 2018.

92 **had a sympathetic animal:** Interview with Celine Minj, January 6, 2018.

92 **Lazarus developed a high fever:** Interview with Celine Minj, January 5, 2018.

93 **Mariana was at the mercy:** Interview with Celine Minj, January 5, 2018.

94 **"I want to study":** Interview with Celine Minj, January 5, 2018.

94 **recognize Celine by the mark:** Interview with Celine Minj, January 5, 2018.

95 **the nursing staff:** Interview with Celine Minj, January 5, 2018.

96 **some new sisters coming:** Interview with Celine Minj, January 5, 2018.

EPIGRAPH

97 **"Amid the wreckage":** Ramachandra Guha, *India After Gandhi: The History of the World's Largest Democracy* (New York: HarperCollins, 2007), 13.

SEVEN: THE OPENING OF NAZARETH HOSPITAL

99 **across the northeastern edge:** Undated hand-drawn map by Marion Batson, in the Patna Bishop's House Archives.

99 **encased in bamboo scaffolding:** Letter from Lawrencetta Veeneman to her family, December 21, 1947; letter from Lawrencetta Veeneman to the motherhouse, December 16, 1947.

100 **the other nine:** Patricia Kelley, Elaine McCarron, and Rachel Willett, *Impelled by the Love of Christ: Sisters of Charity of Nazareth Kentucky, 1936–1948* (2013), 189. Includes the clinic in Ensley, Alabama, that became a hospital in 1948.

100 **first letter from Mokama:** Letter from Lawrencetta Veeneman to her family, December 21, 1947.

100 **word of indeterminate origin:** Etymology of "godown" from *Merriam–Webster Unabridged Dictionary* and *Oxford English Dictionary*.

100 **"This word is used":** Letter from Lawrencetta Veeneman to her family, March 9, 1952.

100 **a big porch:** Letter from Lawrencetta Veeneman to her family, December 21, 1947; letter from Lawrencetta Veeneman to the motherhouse, December 16, 1947.

101 **their evening routine:** Letter from Ann Roberta Powers to the motherhouse, December 19, 1947; letter from Lawrencetta Veeneman to her family, January 18, 1948.

101 **fifty-one years old:** Biographical records from Sisters of Charity of Nazareth Archival Center.

102 **share the news:** Letter from Lawrencetta Veeneman to her family, April 24, 1947.

102 **once wealthy Louisville family:** Interviews with Ed Veeneman, March 14, 2017; Father Dismas Veeneman, March 28, 2017; and Mary Agnes Hanks, March 17, 2017.

103 **her first postings:** Biographical records from Sisters of Charity of Nazareth Archival Center.

103 **"give Him thanks":** Letter from Lawrencetta Veeneman to her family, April 24, 1947.

104 **woke at 4:50:** Letter from Florence Joseph to the motherhouse, March 30, 1948.

104 **They ate porridge:** Letter from Charles Miriam Holt to the motherhouse, January 20, 1948.

104 **immersed in learning Hindi:** Letters from Lawrencetta to the motherhouse, January 10, 1948, and January 25, 1948; letter from Charles Miriam Holt to the motherhouse, February 6, 1948.

104 **"No bread can be bought":** Letter from Charles Miriam Holt to the motherhouse, January 20, 1948; letter from Lawrencetta Veeneman to the motherhouse, January 18, 1948.

105 **the bricks and plaster:** Annals of the Mokameh Mission, January 1, 1948.

105 **capes and hug-me-tights:** Letter from Lawrencetta Veeneman to her family, December 21, 1947.

105 **a young woman to their doorstep:** Annals of the Mokameh Mission, January 5, 1948.

105 **"a good Catholic girl":** Letter from Lawrencetta Veeneman to the motherhouse, January 13, 1948.

105 **Celine looked at what:** Interviews with Celine Minj, January 5 and 6, 2018.

106 **a bed on the roof:** Annals of the Mokameh Mission, January 5, 1948.

106 **help the sisters with their Hindi:** Interviews with Celine Minj, January 5 and 6, 2018; letter from Lawrencetta Veeneman to the motherhouse, January 13, 1948.

106 **cargo from the *Steel Executive*:** Annals of the Mokameh Mission, January 26, 1948.

106 **"The gharries"—cars and other vehicles:** Letter from Charles Miriam Holt to the motherhouse, February 6, 1948.

107 **sedatives, vitamins, antibiotics:** Letter from Crescentia Wise to the motherhouse, December 25, 1948; Sister Eugenia Muething, *Nazareth Along the Banks of the Ganges, 1947–1990* (New York: Harmony House Publishers, 1997), 9.

107 **saved the packing crates:** Letter from Lawrencetta Veeneman to the motherhouse, February 20, 1949; letter to the motherhouse, November 13, 1948.

107 **equipment and construction material:** Annals of the Mokameh Mission, January 27, 1948.

108 **they chose the name:** Letter from Lawrencetta Veeneman to the motherhouse, April 25, 1948.

108 **Gandhi left his quarters:** Ramachandra Guha, *India After Gandhi: The History of the World's Largest Democracy* (New York: HarperCollins, 2007), 845–47.

108 **"Word was received":** Annals of the Mokameh Mission, January 31, 1948.

108 **the threat of violence:** Ramachandra Guha, *Gandhi: The Years that Changed the World, 1914–1948* (New York: Alfred A. Knopf, 2018), 830–34.

109 **"food, homes, clothes and jobs":** Guha, *Gandhi*, 833.

109 **"As the Bible":** Quoted in Guha, *Gandhi*, 857.

110 **"grand coordinated ceremony":** Guha, *Gandhi*, 859.

110 **gathered at the railway station:** Annals of the Mokameh Mission, February 12, 1948.

110 **"What would become":** Quote from the diary of Malcolm Darling in Guha, *Gandhi*, 864.

111 **sisters opened the dispensary:** Letter from Florence Joseph Sauer to the motherhouse, February 8, 1948.

112 **chafed at the idea:** Letter from Charles Miriam Holt to the motherhouse, December 18, 1947; letter from Lawrencetta Veeneman to the motherhouse, February 21, 1948.

112 **her own trip to Kanpur:** Letter from Lawrencetta Veeneman to the motherhouse, March 6, 1948.

112 **"ticking and table linen":** Letter from Lawrencetta Veeneman to the motherhouse, March 6, 1948.

113 **By their first Easter:** Letter from Florence Joseph Sauer to the motherhouse, March 30, 1948; letter from Charles Miriam Holt to the motherhouse, December 18, 1947.

113 **"as quietly as ever":** Letter from Charles Miriam Holt to the motherhouse, February 6, 1948.

113 **"200-yard dash":** Letter from Charles Miriam Holt to the motherhouse, February 6, 1948.

113 **say their prayers:** Letter from Lawrencetta Veeneman to the motherhouse, February 25, 1948; letter from Charles Miriam Holt to the motherhouse, February 6, 1948.

114 **"I don't understand":** Letter from Florence Joseph Sauer to the motherhouse, February 8, 1948.

114 **"not a single word":** Letter from Crescentia Wise to the motherhouse, March 25, 1948.

115 **"That amused us":** Annals of the Mokameh Mission, February 14, 1948.

115 **"the black bonnet":** Letter from Crescentia Wise to the motherhouse, March 25, 1948.

115 **"We can make our retreat":** Letter from Lawrencetta Veeneman to the motherhouse, February 21, 1948.

116 **Their trip to Darjeeling:** Letter from Lawrencetta Veeneman to the motherhouse, April 24, 1948.

116 **"an abundance of water":** Letter from Lawrencetta Veeneman to the motherhouse, April 24, 1948.

116 **three-word phrases:** Letter from Ann Roberta Powers to the motherhouse, May 30, 1948. The examples are the author's.

116 **six duck eggs:** Annals of the Mokameh Mission, February 2, 1948.

116 **Celine took up her pen:** Letter from Celine Minj to the motherhouse, May 29, 1948.

117 **Lawrencetta and the other sisters:** Letter from Lawrencetta Veeneman to the motherhouse, May 14, 1948.

117 **and placed advertisements:** Letter from Lawrencetta Veeneman to her family, June 13, 1948.

117 **time for planting:** Letter from Lawrencetta Veeneman to her family, July 25, 1948.

118 **"Please redouble your prayers":** Letter from Lawrencetta Veeneman to her family, June 13, 1948.

EIGHT: "HE IS YOUNG, ENERGETIC AND ENTHUSIASTIC"

119 **a young man:** Annals of the Mokameh Mission, July 24, 1948.

119 **"I am only sorry":** Letter from Lawrencetta Veeneman to the motherhouse, July 8, 1948.

119 **He thought fondly:** Interview with Erica Lazaro, August 9, 2017. It would have been unusual to find an Indian doctor in Kabul at that time. It's also possible that the elder Dr. Lazaro was in Kanpur, a military town closer to Eric Lazaro's birthplace in Mathura, India.

121 **"young, energetic and enthusiastic":** Letter from Lawrencetta Veeneman to her family, July 25, 1948.

121 **a letter commissioning a "broad survey":** Report of the Health Survey & Development Committee (Calcutta: Government of India Press, 1946), vol. 1, 1, commonly known as the Bhore Committee Report.

122 **Sir Joseph Bhore:** "Sir J. W. Bhore Dead: Former Administrator," *Times of India*, August 18, 1960, 9; "Tribute to Sir Joseph Bhore and Sir Fazl-i-Husain," *Times of India*, March 5, 1935, 12.

123 **starkest numbers were among children:** Bhore Committee Report, vol. 1, 7–21.

123 **increase the number of doctors:** Bhore Committee Report, vol. 2, 31.

123 **1 doctor for every 6,300:** Bhore Committee Report, vol. 1, 36.

123 **Bhore set a target:** Bhore Committee Report, vol. 2, 31.

123 3 annas per person: "Ten-Year Health Plan for India: Village As Nucleus for Organisation," *Times of India*, December 27, 1945, 3.

124 a staff of thirty-eight people: Bhore Committee Report, vol. 2, 38–42.

124 "A lady doctor": "Ten-Year Health Plan for India," 3; need for women doctors in Bhore Committee Report, vol. 1, 64.

124 "Without this goodwill": "Ten-Year Health Plan for India," 3.

124 greeted with fanfare: "Ten-Year Health Plan for India," 3.

125 Lawrencetta would sometimes weep: Letter from Charles Miriam Holt to the motherhouse, April 25, 1948.

125 throes of a psychotic episode: Letter from Crescentia Wise to the motherhouse, March 25, 1948.

126 she had appendicitis: Annals of the Mokameh Mission, April 19, 1950.

126 census of patients: Annals of the Mokameh Mission, August 7, 1948.

126 adapt their evening routine: Annals of the Mokameh Mission, November 22, 1948.

127 "the jackals' serenades": Letter from Ann Roberta Powers to the motherhouse, January 21, 1948.

127 The sisters took advantage: Annals of the Mokameh Mission, October 23, 1948; letter from Charles Miriam Holt to the motherhouse, November 14, 1948.

127 priests' house for his shower: Annals of the Mokameh Mission, November 17, 1948.

127 hills around Nelson County, Kentucky: Letter from Charles Miriam Holt to the motherhouse, July 22, 1948.

127 They celebrated the first anniversary: Annals of the Mokameh Mission, December 13, 1948.

128 village twice a week: Letter from Crescentia Wise to the motherhouse, December 25, 1948.

128 scene at the hospital: Letter from Lawrencetta Veeneman to the motherhouse, September 10, 1948.

128 status of nursing: Bhore Committee Report, vol. 2, 386–87.

128 about 7,000 nurses: Bhore Committee Report, vol. 1, 40.

128 "in no hospital": Bhore Committee Report, vol. 2, 387.

129 the "deplorable" conditions: Bhore Committee Report, vol. 2, 387.

129 Miriam and then Hilda: Annals of the Mokameh Mission, October 9 and November 1, 1948.

129 there was Miss Macqueen: Annals of the Mokameh Mission, March 2 and April 8, 1950.

129 Sister Mary Kieran: Annals of the Mokameh Mission, March 19 and May 2, 1950.

129 but a compounder: Annals of the Mokameh Mission, July 30, 1949.

129 "We have not found her satisfactory": Annals of the Mokameh Mission, October 5, 1948.

130 "just wearing themselves out": Letter from Lawrencetta Veeneman to the motherhouse, September 10, 1948.

130 a "marvelous help": Annals of the Mokameh Mission, January 17, 1949.

130 Babs Gillard's family: Letter from Mother Ann Sebastian and Mother Bertrand to the motherhouse, January 19, 1949. The order's leadership visited India to see the progress of the Mokameh Mission firsthand.

131 Joe was a gregarious man: Interviews with Erica Lazaro, June 16 and August 9, 2017.

131 Her mother, Muriel Gillard: Interview with Erica Lazaro, June 16 and August 9, 2017.

131 had gone to St. Rita's: Letter to the motherhouse, January 29, 1949.

132 hairdresser and a masseuse: Josephine "Babs" Lazaro obituary, *Jersey Journal*, December 28, 2012.

132 the packing-crate shelves: Letter from Lawrencetta Veeneman to the motherhouse, February 20, 1949.

132 Babs's cousin Marie: Annals of the Mokameh Mission, April 8, 1949. The entry in the Annals lists the name as "Muriel," but this may have been in error, as Babs's cousin's name is Marie Gillard. It's also possible that "Muriel Gillard" is Babs's stepmother Cookie (Marguerite), who was also a distant cousin.

132 Marie spent weeks: Annals of the Mokameh Mission, April 2, 1950.

133 a series of heart attacks: Annals of the Mokameh Mission, March 30, 1949.

133 dachshunds she loved so much: Sister Ann Roberta Powers, SCN, "My Story," July 2005, Sisters of Charity of Nazareth Archival Center.

133 Batson had sent them: Letter from Lawrencetta Veeneman to her family, December 11, 1948.

133 barking and yelping: Interview with Sister Ann Roberta, March 2011.

133 Dr. Lazaro had been trying: Annals of the Mokameh Mission, March 30, 1949.

133 drug to treat dengue fever: Letter from Lawrencetta Veeneman to her family, April 26, 1949.

133 carry her in an "invalid chair": Annals of the Mokameh Mission, April 21, 1949; letter from Charles Miriam Holt to the motherhouse, April 26, 1949.

133 carry her to bed: Annals of the Mokameh Mission, April 21, 1949.

133 "a climax to many": Annals of the Mokameh Mission, July 14, 1949.

134 three Maltese sisters: Annals of the Mokameh Mission, September 14, 1949; letter from Florence Joseph Sauer to the motherhouse, September 18, 1949.

134 returned the next day "quite satisfied": Annals of the Mokameh Mission, September 20, 1949.

134 She arrived in November: Annals of the Mokameh Mission, November 19, 1949.

135 **all the people helping them:** Annals of the Mokameh Mission, December 23, 1949.

135 **recorded an income:** Annals of the Mokameh Mission, December 31, 1949.

136 **the wedding of Dr. Lazaro and Babs Gillard:** Annals of the Mokameh Mission, December 26–28, 1949.

136 **her last letter:** Letter from Lawrencetta Veeneman to her family, December 30, 1949.

NINE: HEARTBREAK

139 **lining up to visit:** Annals of the Mokameh Mission, July 12, 1949.

139 **He made his rounds:** Annals of the Mokameh Mission, March 27, 1950.

139 **Babs's Hindi was better:** Letter to the motherhouse, January 29, 1949.

139 **the doctor's devotion:** Letter from Lawrencetta Veeneman to her family, March 19, 1950.

139 **the priests brought the statue:** Annals of the Mokameh Mission, March 17, 1950.

140 **slept in room 2:** Annals of the Mokameh Mission, January 1950.

140 **a bed that Lawrencetta had given them:** Annals of the Mokameh Mission, April 15, 1950.

140 **The local darzi:** Annals of the Mokameh Mission, March 6, 1950.

140 **forty new metal hospital beds:** Annals of the Mokameh Mission, February 1, 1950.

140 **"very much overworked":** Annals of the Mokameh Mission, February 10, 1950.

140 **The Maltese sisters:** Annals of the Mokameh Mission, March 1, 1950.

140 **only two, Celine Minj and Michael Gaetano:** Annals of the Mokameh Mission, April 3, 1950.

140 **take their preliminary exams:** Annals of the Mokameh Mission, March 20, 1950.

141 **Celine and Michael both passed:** Annals of the Mokameh Mission, June 1, 1950.

141 **pay for an expansion:** Annals of the Mokameh Mission, March 18–19, 1950.

141 **They had come from all over:** Annals of the Mokameh Mission, July 15, 1950.

142 **She set aside:** Annals of the Mokameh Mission, July 10, 1950.

142 **The classes were carefully structured:** Annals of the Mokameh Mission, July 17, 1950.

142 **design the nurses' uniforms:** Annals of the Mokameh Mission, April 18, 1950.

142 **darzi added the nurses' uniforms:** Annals of the Mokameh Mission, September 1950.

142 **The frenetic pace:** Annals of the Mokameh Mission, September 1950.

142 **second-floor rooms:** Annals of the Mokameh Mission, September 18, 1950.

142 wiring the second floor: Annals of the Mokameh Mission, September 20, 1950.

142 The electricity was run: Letters from Lawrencetta Veeneman to her family, March 1 and March 27, 1949.

143 its first five-year plan: Ramachandra Guha, *India After Gandhi: The History of the World's Largest Democracy* (New York: HarperCollins, 2007), 211, 214, 216–17; "Rectifying Economic Disequilibrium Caused by War & Partition," *Times of India*, July 10, 1951, 6.

143 second diesel motor: Annals of the Mokameh Mission, April 8, 1950.

143 There were rumors: Letter to the motherhouse, January 22, 1949; letter from Lawrencetta Veeneman to the motherhouse, November 13, 1948.

143 could take hours: Interview with Samir Bose, August 29, 2017.

144 "A man is busy all day long": Letter from Lawrencetta Veeneman to her family, May 8, 1955.

144 water from a railway tank: Letter to the motherhouse, January 22, 1949.

144 jars for canning: Letter from Lawrencetta Veeneman to her family, September 14, 1951.

144 jute for rope lines: Letter from Lawrencetta Veeneman to her family, April 2, 1952.

144 "we have to make the bricks": Letter from Lawrencetta Veeneman to her family, January 19, 1950.

145 Another wave of refugees: Annals of the Mokameh Mission, April 18 and 20, 1950.

145 Mokama, too, had a refugee camp: Annals of the Mokameh Mission, April 12, 1950.

145 When the civil surgeon: Annals of the Mokameh Mission, September 4, 1950.

145 telephone poles were installed: Annals of the Mokameh Mission, December 20, 1950.

145 its own phone number: Letter from Lawrencetta Veeneman to her family, September 14, 1951.

146 Babs had suffered a miscarriage: Annals of the Mokameh Mission, May 30, 1950.

146 Dr. Lazaro had decided to leave: Annals of the Mokameh Mission, March 25, 1950.

146 He had received a cable: Annals of the Mokameh Mission, May 10, 1950.

146 "He is a young man": Letter from Lawrencetta Veeneman to her family, June 7, 1950.

146 some snapshots of life: Letter from Florence Joseph Sauer to the Veeneman family, June 13, 1950.

147 He and Babs went to Calcutta: Annals of the Mokameh Mission, June 12 and 15, 1950.

147 hosted a farewell supper: Annals of the Mokameh Mission, June 20, 1950.

147 transferred to Mokama: Annals of the Mokameh Mission, March 23, 1950.

147 "She is very, very lonely": Annals of the Mokameh Mission, June 24, 1950.

147 Ann Roberta records her disappointment: Letter from Ann Roberta Powers to the motherhouse, February 20, 1949.

148 and mastered Hindi: Letter to the motherhouse, January 29, 1949.

148 good use in the bazaar: Letter to the motherhouse, January 22, 1949.

148 Ann Roberta went over to the boys' school: Annals of the Mokameh Mission, September 1950. The entry refers to events in July 1950.

148 news from the bishop: Annals of the Mokameh Mission, September 20, 1950.

148 The order had been in Patna: Letter from Lawrencetta Veeneman to her family, October 25, 1953.

148 started the school in Gaya: Patricia Kelley, *Fifty Monsoons: Ministry of Change Through Women of India* (New York: Harmony House Publishers, 1999), 122.

148 as enemy aliens: Sister Ann Roberta Powers, SCN, "My Story," July 2005, Sisters of Charity of Nazareth Archival Center.

149 The school at Gaya: Annals of the Mokameh Mission, October 3, 1950.

149 a former Masonic lodge: Letter from Lawrencetta Veeneman to her family, December 2, 1950.

149 They waited for Mother Bertrand: Annals of the Mokameh Mission, October 25, 1950.

149 a letter to Lawrencetta from the bishop: Annals of the Mokameh Mission, November 16, 1950.

149 made plans to leave: Annals of the Mokameh Mission, December 5 and 28, 1950.

149 Babs managed on her own: Annals of the Mokameh Mission, September 4, 1950.

149 She taught the youngest: Letter from Lawrencetta Veeneman to her family, July 31, 1951.

150 Dr. Lazaro found another position: Letter from Lawrencetta Veeneman to her family, March 18, 1951.

150 a bungalow for the young couple: Letter from Lawrencetta Veeneman to her family, January 5, 1952.

150 constant shortages of cement: Letters from Lawrencetta Veeneman to her family, March 12, 1953, and May 28, 1954.

150 "We hope to have the house": Letter from Lawrencetta Veeneman to her family, April 2, 1952.

150 "Babs has at last": Letter from Lawrencetta Veeneman to her family, March 12, 1953.

150 **plans to visit:** Letter from Lawrencetta Veeneman to her family, June 18, 1953.

150 **named chief resident:** Letter from Lawrencetta Veeneman to her family, July 20, 1953.

150 **their little girl arrived:** Letter from Lawrencetta Veeneman to her family, January 30, 1954.

TEN: THE FRONTIER WOMEN OF MOKAMA

151 **lack of electricity:** Annals of the Mokameh Mission, January 1950.

151 **she figured out a way:** Patricia Kelley, *Fifty Monsoons: Ministry of Change Through Women of India* (New York: Harmony House Publishers, 1999), 82–83.

151 **She added a sink:** Annals of the Mokameh Mission, December 1, 1950.

152 **Born Florence Rose Wise:** Biographical records from Sisters of Charity of Nazareth Archival Center.

152 **simple comforts of that life:** Interview with Dolores Vittitow, August 22, 2017.

153 **first of two women:** Kelley, *Fifty Monsoons*, 42.

153 **for the annual meeting:** Sister Crescentia Wise, "The Pharmacist and Parenteral Solutions," presented before Section on Practical Pharmacy and Dispensing, A. Ph. A., New York meeting, 1937, and published June 1938, https://doi.org /10.1002/jps.3080270612.

153 **then set up a still:** Kelley, *Fifty Monsoons*, 82–83.

153 **empty wine bottles:** Letter from Crescentia Wise to the motherhouse, February 20, 1949.

154 **the civil surgeon's visit:** Annals of the Mokameh Mission, September 4, 1950.

154 **patients with leprosy:** Bhore Committee Report, vol. 1, 117, 120.

154 **"He even offers us a leper home":** Sister Eugenia Muething, *Nazareth Along the Banks of the Ganges, 1947–1990* (Harmony House Publishers, 1997), 1.

155 **soon after the dispensary:** Kelley, *Fifty Monsoons*, 87–90.

155 **the hospital's supply:** Annals of the Mokameh Mission, November 11, 1949.

155 **waiting for customs clearance in Bombay:** Annals of the Mokameh Mission, March 21, 1950.

155 **travel for free to Mokama:** Kelley, *Fifty Monsoons*, 85; Muething, *Nazareth on the Banks of the Ganges*, 19.

156 **began in the summer of 1952:** Details of the clinic in Annals of the Mokameh Mission, August 27, 1952; letter from Lawrencetta Veeneman to the motherhouse, June 6, 1953; interview with Bridget Kappalumakal, June 20, 2017.

156 **His name was Ram Dham:** Kathleen Elgin, *Nun: A Gallery of Sisters* (New York: Random House, 1964), 76–77.

156 gathered every Wednesday: Letter from Lawrencetta Veeneman to her family, September 13, 1953.

156 She set up a system: Elgin, *Nun*, 76–77; letter from Mary Martha Wiss to her family, July 28, 1960.

156 Those who arrived: Letter from Lawrencetta Veeneman to the motherhouse, June 6, 1953.

157 treating 625 patients: Annals of the Mokameh Mission, November 25, 1953.

157 more than 1,000: Patna Mission newsletter, December 8, 1953, in the collection of Lawrencetta Veeneman letters.

157 donations of medicine and cash: Annals of the Mokameh Mission, June 21, 29, and 30, 1953.

157 Fulton J. Sheen: Annals of the Mokameh Mission, January 8, 1955.

158 Born Martha Curran: Biographical records from Sisters of Charity of Nazareth Archival Center.

158 a grocery store: Curran family details in letter from Therese Larkin to author, July 2017.

158 a premature baby: Annals of the Mokameh Mission, July 21, 1950.

158 right in the middle: Letter from Therese Larkin to author, July 2017.

159 letters she wrote home: Letter from Ann Cornelius Curran to her father, August 9, 1966.

160 some baffling news: Annals of the Mokameh Mission, January 1, 1954.

160 "When she left": Interview with Sister Patricia Kelley, September 2006, quoted in the biography of Ann Cornelius from Sisters of St. Joseph the Worker.

160 She boarded a plane: Annals of the Mokameh Mission, January 10, 1954.

161 The next morning: Interview with Sister Patricia Kelley, September 2006, quoted in the biography of Ann Cornelius.

161 she has returned "home": Annals of the Mokameh Mission, January 21, 1954.

ELEVEN: THE MAKING OF A LADY DOCTOR

163 a visit to the Veeneman family: Letter from Lawrencetta Veeneman to her family, November 24, 1953.

163 had completed medical school: Letter from Lawrencetta Veeneman to her family, July 20, 1953.

163 "An energetic young woman": Tom Karsell, "First Sister of Charity to Become Physician Completes Four-Year Residency in Surgery," (Louisville) *Courier-Journal*, July 5, 1958.

163 replacements for Dr. Lazaro: Letter from Lawrencetta Veeneman to her family, May 6, 1951, and October 1, 1953.

164 a succession of substitute doctors: Letter from Lawrencetta Veeneman to her family, August 18, 1952.

164 Dr. Lazaro's classmates: Annals of the Mokameh Mission, June 8, 1950.

164 There was Dr. Gernon: Annals of the Mokameh Mission, June 20, 1950.

164 Then Dr. De Silva: Annals of the Mokameh Mission, August 20, 1950; letter from Lawrencetta Veeneman to her family, July 31, 1951.

164 "All three of these doctors": Letter from Lawrencetta Veeneman to her family, October 1, 1953.

164 replaced by Dr. Smith: Letter from Lawrencetta Veeneman to her family, October 1, 1953.

164 a young Catholic couple: Letter from Lawrencetta Veeneman to her family, October 25, 1953.

164 then came Dr. D'Cruze: Letter from Mary Martha Wiss to her family, July 28, 1959.

165 the hospital in India was "completely different": Letter from Ann Cornelius to the motherhouse, May 7, 1948.

165 "She has let me do": Letter from Crescentia Wise to the motherhouse, July 11, 1948.

166 centuries of patriarchal notions: Katherine Burton, *According to the Pattern: The Story of Dr Agnes McLaren and the Society of Catholic Medical Missionaries* (New York: Longmans Green & Co, 1946), 90–91, 96–100, 108–10; Ailish Veale, "International and Modern Ideals in Irish Female Medical Missionary Activity, 1937–1962," *Women's History Review* 25, no. 4 (2016): 602–18, DOI:10.1080/09612025.2015.1114330.

166 lack of medical care available to women: Burton, *According to the Pattern*, 86–89.

166 established St. Catherine's Hospital: Burton, *According to the Pattern*, 100.

166 women suffered or died: Burton, *According to the Pattern*, 93. The author quotes the Indian writer Pundita Ramabai Sarasvati, who observed that the greatest defect in India was the lack of women doctors: "The want of them is the cause of hundreds of thousands of women dying prematurely."

167 to train a religious community: Burton, *According to the Pattern*, 108–9.

167 traveled to Rome five times: Burton, *According to the Pattern*, 118.

167 a young Austrian woman: Burton, *According to the Pattern*, 122–23.

167 her mentor's work in Rawalpindi: Burton, *According to the Pattern*, 153.

168 "publicly" professed sisters: Burton, *According to the Pattern*, 216.

168 *Constans ac Sedula*: Burton, *According to the Pattern*, 213–15.

168 different orders interpreted it differently: October 11, 2019, email communication with Dr. Carmen M. Mangion, Department of History, Classics, and Archaeology, Birkbeck, University of London; see also Barbra Mann Wall, *Unlikely*

Entrepreneurs: Catholic Sisters and the Hospital Marketplace, 1865–1925 (Columbus: Ohio State University Press, 2005).

168 "It was church law": Karsell, "First Sister of Charity to Become Physician."

168 played the violin beautifully: Interviews with Margaret Thornton, March and May 2017.

169 "it was a big decision for me": Karsell, "First Sister of Charity to Become Physician."

169 "I was waiting for the chance": Karsell, "First Sister of Charity to Become Physician."

169 Mary had been fascinated: William Lynwood Montell, *Tales from Kentucky Doctors* (Lexington: University Press of Kentucky, 2008), 20–21.

170 same one where his father and brother: Interview with John Wiss, August 8, 2017.

171 Lucille graduated with two degrees: Interview with John Wiss, August 8, 2017.

172 low-class habits: Interview with Dr. Pauline Fox, March 24, 2017.

173 People told her: From Dale Deaton's interview of Mary Martha Wiss and Pauline Fox, February 14, 1979, for the Frontier Nursing Service Oral History project.

173 She liked the crowd: Montell, *Tales from Kentucky Doctors*, 20–21.

173 Mary Wiss entered the convent: Mary Wiss obituary.

174 she had to wear the habit all through medical school: Interviews with Margaret Thornton, March and May 2017.

174 she used to joke: Interview with Dr. Pauline Fox, March 23, 2017.

175 how to read X-rays: Interview with Dr. Pauline Fox, March 23, 2017.

TWELVE: WOMEN OF THE NEW INDIA

177 their distinctive names: Annals of the Mokameh Mission, January 15, 1951.

177 Anglo-Indians began to leave: Mian Ridge, "Fadeout for a Culture That's Neither Indian nor British," *New York Times*, August 14, 2010.

177 a new class of fourteen: Annals of the Mokameh Mission, July 9, 1954.

177 from parish priests: Annals of the Mokameh Mission, April 25, 1950; interviews with Bridget Kappalumakal, June 2017. Sebastian Pinakat was an especially influential parish priest who encouraged many young women from Kerala who wanted to leave home to become nuns or nurses.

178 storied community of Indian Catholics: from A. K. Gopalan, *Kerala Past and Present* (London: Lawrence & Wishart, 1959), 22–25.

178 a natural choice: Annals of the Mokameh Mission, March 30, 1950.

178 Three of the sisters: Letter to the motherhouse, November 27, 1947.

178 Christians from the Middle East: Sonja Thomas, *Privileged Minorities: Syrian Christianity, Gender, and Minority Rights in Postcolonial India* (Seattle: University of Washington Press, 2018), 4, 5.

179 **about 40 percent:** Thomas, *Privileged Minorities*, 27.

179 **decided to make their case:** Annals of the Mokameh Mission, November and December 1954.

179 **An account of their trip:** Patricia Kelley, *Fifty Monsoons: Ministry of Change Through Women of India* (New York: Harmony House Publishers, 1999), 147–49.

179 **"They explained to the girls":** Kelley, *Fifty Monsoons*, 147–49.

180 **One of them was Bridget Kappalumakal:** Her biography from interviews with Bridget Kappalumakal, June 2017; see also Kelly McDaniels, "Sister Bridget Kappalumakal: A Profile," published online by the Sisters of Charity of Nazareth, September 26, 2018, https://scnfamily.org/sister-bridget-kappalumakal-a-profile/.

184 **their position of privilege:** Ramachandra Guha, *India After Gandhi: The History of the World's Largest Democracy* (New York: HarperCollins, 2007), 296–300.

185 **Rose was one of these girls:** Rose's biography from interviews in April and May 2017. Rose asked not to be identified by her name. I have changed it at her request, and some identifying details.

EPIGRAPH

193 **"What, then is the use":** Ruth Prawer Jhabvala, *The Nature of Passion: A Novel* (New York: W. W. Norton, 1957), 153.

THIRTEEN: THE NOVICES GO ON STRIKE

195 **hospital received its first phone call:** Letter from Lawrencetta Veeneman to her family, September 14, 1951; Annals of the Mokameh Mission, July 27 and August 6, 1951.

195 **rural electricity finally reached Mokama:** Letter from Lawrencetta Veeneman to her family, December 10, 1955; Annals of the Mokameh Mission, October 30, 1955, and April 1956.

196 **piped running water:** Annals of the Mokameh Mission, January 8 and April 13, 1957.

196 **Mokama was designated as a "Notified Area":** Annals of the Mokameh Mission, March 29, 1955.

196 **shipments sent to Mokama:** Annals of the Mokameh Mission, March 1952.

196 **a meeting in Calcutta:** Annals of the Mokameh Mission, August 8, August 16, and September 23, 1952.

196 **in 1955, UNICEF:** Annals of the Mokameh Mission, July 10, 1955.

196 **Bridget's group of five:** Interviews with Bridget Kappalumakal, June 2017; Annals of the Mokameh Mission, July 9, 1955.

197 **"Yes, we will start a novitiate":** Letter from Lawrencetta Veeneman to her family, October 14, 1954.

197 "for the clothing ceremony": Annals of the Mokameh Mission, April 9, 1951.

198 "native orders" of Catholic sisters: Annals of the Mokameh Mission, August and October 1952, February 3, 1953.

198 "looked like little dolls": Letter from Lawrencetta Veeneman to her family, December 10, 1955.

198 Bridget's class—stayed in the same dormitory: Interviews with Bridget Kappalumakal, June 2017.

199 one of the nurses asked Bridget: Interviews with Bridget Kappalumakal, June 2017.

201 46,000 textile workers: "General Strike Starts," *Times of India*, May 3, 1955, 11; "Indian Strike Sets Record," *New York Times*, July 4, 1955.

201 Workers in Bombay: "India Mobs Riot over Goa Deaths," *New York Times*, August 17, 1955, 1.

201 Portugal had troops in Goa: Ramachandra Guha, *India After Gandhi: The History of the World's Largest Democracy* (New York: HarperCollins, 2007), 184–86.

201 sister who came to stay with them: Annals of the Mokameh Mission, August 17, 1955.

202 Bridget and the others all passed: Annals of the Mokameh Mission, April 3, 1956.

202 already made an application: Letter from Lawrencetta Veeneman to her family, January 5, 1956.

202 "we know the vocations will come": Letter from Lawrencetta Veeneman to her family, January 5, 1956.

202 Mother Bertrand asked the vicar general: Patricia Kelley, *Fifty Monsoons: Ministry of Change Through Women of India* (New York: Harmony House Publishers, 1999), 149.

202 "We need some recruits": Letter from Lawrencetta Veeneman to her family, April 29, 1956.

203 started work on expanding the chapel: Letter from Lawrencetta Veeneman to her family, May 21, 1956.

203 She immediately went to Lawrencetta: Account of the strike in Kelley, *Fifty Monsoons*, 151–52; interviews with Bridget Kappalumakal, June 2017.

204 made her first recruiting trip: Letter from Lawrencetta Veeneman to her family, December 13, 1956; Annals of the Mokameh Mission December 26, 1956, and January 12, 1957; details of the trip in letters from Lawrencetta Veeneman to her family, January 1 and January 28, 1957.

204 mistress of novices: Letter from Lawrencetta Veeneman to her family, October 20, 1956; Annals of the Mokameh Mission September 8, 1956.

205 only two candidates: Annals of the Mokameh Mission, January 13, 1957.

205 her last night in Champakulam: Letter from Lawrencetta Veeneman to her family, January 28, 1957.

206 her size 10½ feet: Letter from Lawrencetta Veeneman to her family, March 19 and September 18, 1957.

206 begin their novitiate: Kelley, *Fifty Monsoons*, 152; Annals of the Mokameh Mission, February 2, 1957.

206 the five women: Annals of the Mokameh Mission, February 2, 1957.

206 Bridget began the regimented life: Interviews with Bridget Kappalumakal, June 2017; interview with Nirmala Mulackal, August 2016.

207 observe "sacred silence": Interview with Margaret Rodericks, May 2017; interview with Nirmala Mulackal, August 2016.

208 two unmarried sisters: Letters from Lawrencetta Veeneman to her family, August 3, September 12 and 14, 1955.

208 the third, who had died suddenly: Letter from Lawrencetta Veeneman to her family, November 29, 1953.

208 their mother passed away: Letters from Lawrencetta Veeneman to her family, August 3 and August 29, 1953, September 3, 1953.

208 suffered from mental illness: Letters from Lawrencetta Veeneman to her family, April 28 and November 29, 1963.

208 her brother Lawrence: Letters from from sisters Elizabeth Emmanuel and Augustine Marie to the Veeneman family, February 26, 1962.

208 gathered around a large cotton tree: Letter from Lawrencetta Veeneman to her family, April 24, 1960.

208 one special Christmas morning: Annals of the Mokameh Mission, December 25, 1962.

208 Bridget became one of the first: Letter from Lawrencetta Veeneman to her family, December 17, 1957; also in interviews with Bridget Kappalumakal, June 2017; Annals of the Mokameh Mission, December 8, 1957.

208 Bridget submitted to a ritual: Interviews with Bridget Kappalumakal, June 2017.

FOURTEEN: THE ENGLISH-ONLY RULE

211 For Rose, after the relative freedom: Interviews with Rose, March 2016, and April and May 2017.

211 lice and tapeworms: Interviews with Rose, March 2016, and April and May 2017; interviews with Elizabeth and Elsamma Thottam, 2016 and 2017.

211 Rose found it difficult: Interviews with Rose, March 2016, and April and May 2017.

212 "American" way to wash dishes: Author's reporting.

212 sat with the others and talked in Malayalam: Interviews with Rose, March 2016, and April and May 2017.

212 Leela had come to Mokama: Interview with Leela Thomas, March 2016.

213 Elizabeth, the schoolteacher's daughter: Interview with Elizabeth, March 2016. I have identified her only as "Elizabeth," at her request.

213 Elsy, one of the girls who had traveled: Interviews with Elsamma Thottam, 2016 and 2017.

214 She had few models: Interviews with Elsamma Thottam, 2016 and 2017.

215 The nuns wouldn't allow them: Interviews with Rose, March 2016, and April and May 2017; interviews with Elizabeth, March 2016, and Elsamma Thottam, 2016 and 2017.

215 inserted chewing tobacco: Interview with Betty Howell, April 2016.

215 Celine Minj, who had become a supervisor: Interview with Celine Minj, January 6, 2018.

216 given fourteen uniforms: Interview with Celine Minj, January 6, 2018.

216 Celine demonstrated how: Interviews with Celine Minj, January 6, 2018.

216 Celine showed them how to manage: Interviews with Celine Minj, January 6, 2018; interviews with Rose, March 2016, and April and May 2017.

217 nothing like this cold in Kerala: Interview with Betty Howell, April 2016.

217 Florence Joseph, who had taken over: Annals of the Mokameh Mission, September 8, 1956.

217 Florence Joseph was a farmer's daughter: Death certificate for John Joseph Sauer; biographical records from Sisters of Charity of Nazareth Archival Center; 1930 and 1940 census records; findagrave.com records for Sauer family.

218 Florence Joseph was only thirty-seven years old: Biographical records from Sisters of Charity of Nazareth Archival Center; appointed superior, September 8, 1956.

218 Her voice carried: Interviews with Gail Collins, July 2016, and Nirmala Mulackal.

218 She once went to a ten-day meeting: Annals of the Mokameh Mission, March 15, 1964; interview with Gail Collins, July 2016.

219 "Yes, we should do this": Interview with Gail Collins, July 2016.

219 she raised thousands of rupees: Annals of the Mokameh Mission, February 13 and June 14, 1961.

219 To the student nurses: Interviews with Rose, March 2016, and April and May 2017; interview with Leela Thomas, March 2016; interviews with Elizabeth, March 2016, and Elsamma Thottam, 2016 and 2017.

219 patrol the dormitory: Interviews with Rose, March 2016, and April and May 2017; interview with Leela Thomas, March 2016; interviews with Elizabeth, March 2016, and Elsamma Thottam, 2016 and 2017.

220 homesick, especially for rice: Interview with Leela Thomas, March 2016.

220 Leela finally had enough: Interview with Leela Thomas, March 2016.

221 knocked her into a ditch: Annals of the Mokameh Mission, February 15, 1953.

222 Ann Cornelius had her favorites: Interviews with Rose, March 2016, and April and May 2017; interview with Leela Thomas, March 2016; interviews with Elizabeth, March 2016, and Elsamma Thottam, 2016 and 2017.

222 Crescentia was more fun: Interviews with Rose, March 2016, and April and May 201; interview with Leela Thomas, March 2016.

222 One incident became legendary: Interviews with Rose, March 2016, and April and May 2017; interview with Leela Thomas, March 2016; interviews with Elizabeth, March 2016, and Elsamma Thottam, 2016 and 2017.

223 high school diplomas: Interviews with Rose, March 2016, and April and May 2017; interview with Leela Thomas, March 2016; interviews with Elizabeth, March 2016, and Elsamma Thottam, 2016 and 2017.

223 By 1955, language had come to define: A thorough account of the reorganization of India's states by language in Ramachandra Guha, *India After Gandhi: The History of the World's Largest Democracy* (New York: HarperCollins, 2007), 189–208.

224 "not only a binding force": Guha, *India After Gandhi*, 192, quoting JVP committee.

224 the death by fasting: Guha, *India After Gandhi*, 197.

224 a trip to Trivandrum: Interview with Elizabeth, March 2016.

225 they would punish them: Interview with Elizabeth, March 2016.

225 Leela was discovered: Interview with Leela Thomas, March 2016.

226 did not charge any fees: Interviews with Rose, March 2016, and April and May 2017; interview with Leela Thomas, March 2016; interviews with Elsamma Thottam, 2016 and 2017.

227 There was Aleykutty: Annals of the Mokameh Mission, November 13, 1962.

227 the girl who scandalized: Interview with Rose, March 2016, and April and May 2017; interview with Leela Thomas, March 2016; interviews with Elsamma Thottam, 2016 and 2017.

227 parents in Kerala: Letter from Lawrencetta Veenaman to her family, August 24, 1965.

228 Leela, in the end, won her appeal: Interview with Leela Thomas, March 2016.

228 Chedilal's sari shop: Interview with Betty Howell, April 2016.

228 Elizabeth was so proud: Interview with Elizabeth, March 2016.

229 their favorite place: Interview with Elizabeth, March 2016.

229 had bought bicycles: Letter from Mary Martha Wiss to her family, December 11, 1960.

FIFTEEN: MISS WISS AND DR. KENNY

231 more than a year before: Letter to the motherhouse, August 1957.

231 twenty-three boxes of cargo: Annals of the Mokameh Mission, August 12 and 14, 1958.

231 **more than six hundred dollars:** Letter from Mary Martha Wiss to her family, April 21, 1959.

231 **Dr. Meave Kenny:** Annals of the Mokameh Mission, August 3, 1958, and March 29, 1959.

232 **boarded the S.S.** *Steel Navigator*: Letter from Mary Martha Wiss to her family, March 15, 1959.

232 **Dr. Wiss arrived in India:** Annals of the Mokameh Mission, April 14, 1959.

232 **the bridge across the Ganges:** Letter from Mary Martha Wiss to her family, June 27, 1959.

232 **Dr. Kenny supervised:** Letter from Mary Martha Wiss to her family, July 28, 1959.

232 **Dr. D'Cruze interrupted:** Letter from Mary Martha Wiss to her family, July 19, 1959.

232 **"This is really a huge bridge":** Letter from Mary Martha Wiss to her family, August 9, 1959.

233 **the previous day's activity:** Letter from Mary Martha Wiss to her family, July 12, 1959.

233 **forty-eight cases in a week:** Letter from Mary Martha Wiss to her family, August 9, 1959.

234 **Dr. Wiss complained:** Letter from Mary Martha Wiss to Captain Robert L. Reid, January 14, 1960. The letter refers to his "residency," so he may have been a fellow surgical resident at St. Joseph's.

234 **operating-room light bulbs:** Letter from Mary Martha Wiss to her family, June 27, 1959.

234 **lack of an X-ray machine:** Letter from Mary Martha Wiss to her family, July 19, 1959.

234 **range of medical problems:** Letter from Mary Martha Wiss to her family, October 25, 1959.

234 **anemia and other illnesses:** Letters from Mary Martha Wiss to her family, November 15 and 22, 1959.

234 **eight-year-old girl:** Letter from Mary Martha Wiss to her family, July 5, 1959.

234 **nearly lost his foot:** Letters from Mary Martha Wiss to her family, December 20, 1959, and January 9 and June 19, 1960.

234 **fifteen-pound dermoid cyst:** Letter from Mary Martha Wiss to her family, May 8, 1960.

234 **falling from a tree:** Letter from Mary Martha Wiss to her family, June 10, 1963.

235 **a glowing profile:** "S is for Sister and also Surgeon," *Ohio State University Monthly*, November 1959, 11.

235 **"a wonderful dream come true":** Nazareth Hospital Christmas card, December 25, 1959, sent by Lawrencetta Veeneman to her family.

235 **"the change is tremendous"**: Letter from Mary Martha Wiss to the motherhouse, September 24, 1959.

236 **"subtotal resection of the stomach"**: Letter from Mary Martha Wiss to her family, September 13, 1959.

236 **The four-year-old son**: Letter from Mary Martha Wiss to her family, September 13, 1959.

236 **her favorite operas and symphonies**: Letter from Mary Martha Wiss to her family, September 5 and 13, 1959.

236 **already had a heart attack**: Interview with Margaret Thornton, March 30, 2017.

237 **reproduce them by mimeograph**: Letters from Mary Martha Wiss to her family, August 9 and October 25, 1959.

237 **"the readers of this epistle"**: Letter from Mary Martha Wiss to her family, October 11, 1959.

237 **"our big white concrete building"**: Detailed descriptions in letter from Mary Martha Wiss to her family, September 24, 1959, and letter from Mary Martha Wiss to Johnny Wiss, July 31, 1959.

238 **own set of tools**: Letter from Mary Martha Wiss to her family, February 6, 1959.

238 **set up makeshift traction**: Interview with Rose, March 22, 2016.

238 **repairs to the phonograph**: Letter from Mary Martha Wiss to her family, June 18 and October 11, 1959.

238 **six-inch wrench**: Letter from Mary Martha Wiss to her family, May 8 and December 18, 1960.

238 **plaster of Paris**: Letter from Mary Martha Wiss to her family, May 8, 1960.

238 **a new method to treat babies born with clubfoot**: Letter from Mary Martha Wiss to her family, February 4, 1961.

238 **The Bata shoe factory**: Letter from Mary Martha Wiss to her family, December 27, 1959.

239 **but industrial accidents**: Letter from Mary Martha Wiss to her family, May 29, 1960.

239 **The Barauni refinery**: Letters from Mary Martha Wiss to her family, February 11 and March 10, 1962.

239 **the four-month-old baby boy**: Letter from Mary Martha Wiss to her family, July 28, 1960.

239 **The girl with the severely burned hand**: Letters from Mary Martha Wiss to her family, September 26 and October 3, 1959.

240 **the annual Durga Puja festival**: Letter from Mary Martha Wiss to her family, October 18, 1959.

240 **"Dr. Kenny can do"**: Letter from Mary Martha Wiss to her family, September 13, 1959.

241 "learned a little more about Dr. Kenny": Letter from Mary Martha Wiss to her family, September 13, 1959.

241 exaggerated surgical saw: Letter from Mary Martha Wiss to her family, undated, 1959.

242 as "gentlemen's plumber": The phrase is in letter from Mary Martha Wiss to her family, November 3, 1962; more on Kenny's work in infertility clinic is in letter from Mary Martha Wiss to her family, November 7, 1959.

242 called the doctor "Miss Wiss": Letter from Sister Eugenia to the Wiss family, September 13, 1959.

242 "may have a cobra skin": Letters from Mary Martha Wiss to her family, January 9 and June 27, 1960.

242 swear words in Hindi in the bazaar: Letter from Mary Martha Wiss to her family, November 8, 1960.

242 pick up a birdbath: Letter from Mary Martha Wiss to her family, October 18, 1959.

242 record her lectures: Letter from Mary Martha Wiss to her family, November 1, 1959.

242 a love for animals: Letters from Mary Martha Wiss to her family, November 7 and December 2, 1959, and January 29, May 1, and June 12, 1960.

243 boarding school in Darjeeling: Letter from Mary Martha Wiss to her family, March 5, 1960.

243 borrowed a couple of horses: Letter from Mary Martha Wiss to her family, January 31, 1960.

243 an afternoon "spree": Letter from Mary Martha Wiss to her family, December 18, 1960.

243 Flossie and Joey: Letter from Dr. Kenny to the Wiss family, February 14, 1960.

243 Dr. Kenny wrote directly to the Wiss family: Letter from Dr. Kenny to the Wiss family, February 14, 1960.

243 could work on their correspondence: Letter from Mary Martha Wiss to her family, May 29, 1960.

244 an uncensored letter: Letter from Mary Martha Wiss to her family, November 19, 1959.

244 resent the success: Mention of doctors trying to discredit them in the bazaar in Annals of the Mokameh Mission, May 9, 1950; letters from Mary Martha Wiss to her family, May 15 and September 25, 1960.

244 lost her patience: Letter from Mary Martha Wiss to her family, October 10, 1960.

245 "Don't forget that": Letter from Mary Martha Wiss to her family, November 19, 1959.

245 **case of allergic dermatitis:** Letter from Mary Martha Wiss to her family, September 26, 1959.

245 **gloves made of neoprene:** Letters from Mary Martha Wiss to her family, November 15 and December 1, 1959.

245 **She was elected president:** From photograph of the "Mokameh Branch of the I.M.A., 1960–61," presumably the Indian Medical Association.

246 **planned to leave India:** Departure in Annals of the Mokameh Mission, February 28, 1961; letter from Dr. Kenny to Mr. and Mrs. Wiss, November 10, 1960.

246 **a new suitcase:** Letter from Mary Martha Wiss to her family, November 8, 1960.

246 **one more letter to the Wiss family:** Letter from Dr. Kenny to the Wiss family, November 10, 1960.

246 **"Well, we've had a good year":** Letter from Dr. Kenny to the Wiss family, November 10, 1960.

SIXTEEN: THE FLOOD

249 **The rains began:** Letter from Lawrencetta Veeneman to her family, October 11, 1961; account of the flood also in Annals of the Mokameh Mission, October 1, 1961.

250 **It was a week:** Letter from Lawrencetta Veeneman to her family, October 11, 1961; account of the flood also in Annals of the Mokameh Mission, October 1, 1961.

250 **Sister Ann Cornelius had gone:** Letter from Lawrencetta Veeneman to her family, October 11, 1961; account of the flood also in Annals of the Mokameh Mission, October 1, 1961.

251 **Dr. Wiss had gone to Madras:** Letter from Mary Martha Wiss to her family, October 5, 1961; more details in letter from Mary Martha Wiss to her family, October 13, 1961.

251 **her patient, Sister James Leo:** Annals of the Mokameh Mission, September 21, 1961.

251 **assessed the damage:** Details on the Bihar floods of 1961 from newspaper accounts: "Bihar Floods Exact Toll of Nearly 900 Human Lives," *Times of India*, October 10, 1961, 1; "Flood Toll in Bihar Has Risen to 908," *Times of India*, October 11, 1961, 1; "15,000-Sq.-Mile Area Floods in Bihar," *Times of India*, October 7, 1961, 1; "Four-Day Deluge Ends," *Times of India* News Service, October 5, 1961, 1; "Hundreds Killed in Bihar Floods," *Times of India*, October 8, 1961, 1; "The Battered Face of Bihar," *Times of India*, October 22, 1961, 9; "Nehru May Survey Flood Damage," *Times of India*, October 11, 1961, 1.

252 **perhaps a thousand or more:** "Bihar Dead Put at 1,000," *New York Times*, October 10, 1961.

252 **These lowlands extend:** Letter from Lawrencetta Veeneman to her family, August 19, 1951.

252 **taal land is different from diara land:** Interview with Ashok Anshuman, January 2018; interview with Ajay Kumar January 2018; Sumitap Ranjan et al., "Assessment of Soil Fertility of Tal and Diara Land: A Case Study of Bhagalpur District, Bihar, India," *Journal of Pharmacognosy and Phytochemistry* 7, no. 5 (2018): 1178–80, https://www.phytojournal.com/archives/2018/vol7issue5/PartU/7-5-200-500.pdf.

252 **When the water recedes:** Description in letter to the motherhouse, January 29, 1949.

253 **bhumihars of Mokama:** Interviews with Ajay Kumar and Venkatesh Narayan Singh, January 2018.

254 **the legend of Reshma and Chuharmal:** For a detailed analysis of the myth, see Badri Narayan, *Documenting Dissent: Contesting Fables, Contested Minorities and Dalit Political Discourse* (Shimla: Indian Institute of Advanced Study, 2001), 23–51.

254 **Mokama held a fair:** Narayan, *Documenting Dissent*, 35–39, 50–51.

255 **They owned almost everything:** Interview with Venkatesh Narayan Singh, January 2018.

255 **Mokama's one cinema hall:** Letter from Mary Martha Wiss to her family, November 7, 1959.

255 **refused to allow a popular film:** Interview with Ajay Kumar, January 2018.

255 **lived in a traditional home:** Author reporting on visit to this home.

256 **the children chafed:** Interview with Ajay Kumar, January 2018.

257 **knew the American women:** Interviews with Ajay Kumar and Venkatesh Narayan Singh, January 2018.

258 **"Bibhuthi, the grandson":** Annals of the Mokameh Mission, July 26, 1961.

258 **there were fifty-five deaths:** Annals of the Mokameh Mission, "Nazareth Hospital, Mokameh Junction, January 1, 1961–December 31, 1961"; total deaths in this period recorded in an undated entry (most likely January 1, 1962) summarizing the year.

259 **He came to the hospital in a rage:** Interview with archivist at Nazareth Hospital and Convent, Mokama, July 2016.

259 **dismissed the lawsuit:** Letter from Mary Martha Wiss to her family, September 3, 1961.

259 **"The 'Case' was to have been convened":** Annals of the Mokameh Mission, January 25, 1962.

259 **Florence Joseph proudly noted:** Letter from Florence Joseph Sauer to the Wiss family, May 27, 1961.

260 **white Leghorn chickens:** Letter from Lawrencetta Veeneman to her family, January 29, 1961.

260 rumors that circulated about them: Annals of the Mokameh Mission, May 9, 1950. As early as 1950, the sisters worried about the doctors in the bazaar who were trying to discredit them.

260 The lawsuit had been dismissed: Annals of the Mokameh Mission, April 1962.

261 Singh and his family recalled: Interviews with Ajay Kumar and Venkatesh Narayan Singh, January 2018.

SEVENTEEN: ARRIVALS

263 In the spring of 1963: Letter from Mary Martha Wiss to her family, March 11, 1963.

263 graduating from West Point: Interviews with Margaret Thornton and John Wiss, 2017.

263 born on the same day: Interviews with Margaret Thornton and John Wiss, 2017; John Wiss obituary.

263 she fell ill: Letter from Mary Martha Wiss to her family, January 30, 1963; Annals of the Mokameh Mission, January 3–5, 1963.

263 a doctor from the Medical Missionaries: Letters from Mary Martha Wiss to her family, February 10, 24, and 27, 1963.

264 "as some sort of crisis": Letter from Mary Martha Wiss to her family, March 11, 1963.

264 Johnny had found a way: Letter from Mary Martha Wiss to her family, March 11, 1963.

264 Nehru summoned Ambassador Galbraith: Ramachandra Guha, *India After Gandhi: The History of the World's Largest Democracy* (New York: HarperCollins, 2007), 337.

265 another uncensored letter home: Letter from Mary Martha Wiss to her family, November 4, 1962.

265 a thousand rupees in cash: Annals of the Mokameh Mission, November 17 and 20, 1962.

265 a lecture later that month: Annals of the Mokameh Mission, November 24, 1962.

265 "two major operations": Annals of the Mokameh Mission, March 16, 1963.

266 new Russian oil refinery: Guha, *India After Gandhi*, 219; letters from Mary Martha Wiss to her family, February 11 and March 10, 1962.

266 learned enough Russian: Letters from Mary Martha Wiss to her family, June 6, 1962, and July 27, 1963.

266 a few days together: Letter from Lawrencetta Veeneman to her family, March 26, 1963; Annals of the Mokameh Mission, March 18–30, 1963.

266 Johnny made himself useful: Letter from John Wiss to his family, March 29, 1963; letter from Mary Jude to the Wiss family, March 30, 1963.

267 **Jackie Kennedy's personal physician:** Letter from Mary Jude to the Wiss family, April 4, 1963.

267 **the two other older sisters:** Departure of Charles Miriam Holt in letter from Lawrencetta Veeneman to her family, May 8, 1961; permanent departure of Crescentia, letter from Lawrencetta Veeneman to her family, May 31, 1962.

267 **Pope Paul VI:** Xavier Rynne, "Letter from Vatican City," *New Yorker*, December 25, 1965.

268 **The council had opened:** Rynne, "Letter from Vatican City."

268 **"looking outward and looking inward":** John W. O'Malley, *What Happened at Vatican II* (Cambridge, MA: Harvard University Press, 2010), 317.

268 **a simple veil:** Annals of the Mokameh Mission, October 29, 1963; letter from Lawrencetta Veeneman to her family, April 29, 1956.

268 **they kept up:** Letter from Lawrencetta Veeneman to her family, November 12, 1962.

269 **something of a celebrity:** Letter from Lawrencetta Veeneman to her family, November 12, 1962.

269 **years earlier on a trip to Bombay:** Letter from Lawrencetta Veeneman to her family, December 1955.

269 **the shortage of nurses:** Letter to Lawrencetta Veeneman from her sister Lucy, January 21, 1960.

269 **permission to write home:** Letter from Lawrencetta Veeneman to her family, March 19, 1961.

270 **permission to visit her family:** Letters from Lawrencetta Veeneman to her family, May 15 and July 7, 1963.

270 **Her return to Mokama:** Annals of the Mokameh Mission, September 3, 1963.

271 **back at full speed in the operating room:** Letter from Mary Martha Wiss to her family, February 20, 1964; Annals of the Mokameh Mission, February 10, 1964.

271 **volvulus, or twisting, of the lower colon:** Letter from Mary Martha Wiss to her family, July 4, 1964.

271 **Mary Martha was impatient:** Letters from Mary Martha Wiss to her family, June 27, 1963, and February 23, 1964.

271 **"One of my stock":** Letter from Mary Martha Wiss to her family, September 22, 1963.

272 **"The leading families":** Letter from Mary Martha Wiss to her family, February 23, 1964.

272 **the Eucharistic Congress:** "Cardinal Opens Bombay Congress: 100,000 People Assemble for Eucharistic Session," *New York Times*, November 29, 1964, https://www.nytimes.com/1964/11/29/archives/cardial-opens-bombay -congress-100000-people-assemble-for.html.

272 **pay for her airfare to Bombay:** Letters from Lawrencetta Veeneman to her family, May 4, September 14, and October 18, 1964.

272 **"A FAMILY evening"**: Annals of the Mokameh Mission, July 19, 1964.

273 **Mary Martha took ill**: Annals of the Mokameh Mission, July 26, July 30, and August 15, 1964.

273 **she wrote to her parents with the news**: Letter from Mary Martha Wiss to her family, August 23, 1964.

273 **one of them, Mary Jude**: Letter from Sister Mary Jude to Mr. H. Miller, August 25, 1964, in collection of Wiss letters; letter from Mary Jude to Wiss family, August 26, 1964.

273 **a buzz of activity**: Annals of the Mokameh Mission, August 18 and September 9, 10, 12, and 13, 1964.

274 **her last letter home**: Letter from Mary Martha Wiss to her family, September 3, 1964.

EIGHTEEN: DEPARTURES

275 **The Air India jet from Rome to Bombay**: "Pope Will Fly Tomorrow to Bombay, with Stop at Beirut, to Attend Eucharistic Congress," *New York Times*, December 1, 1964, https://www.nytimes.com/1964/12/02/archives/pope-paul-flies-to-rites-in-india-leaves-by-jet-for-eucharistic.html; "Pope Paul Flies to Rites in India," *New York Times*, December 2, 1964.

275 **More than three hundred thousand people**: For the scene of the visit see newsreel from British Pathé, https://www.youtube.com/watch?v=5Qn__9BqS7U, http://library.stu.edu/ulma/va/3005/1964/12-11-1964.pdf.

275 **Mass, where 3,600 children**: "3600 Children at Rally Receive Communion," 3; "130 Ordained as Priests in Colorful Bombay Rites," 2, *The Voice*, December 11, 1964.

276 **coming as a "pilgrim"**: Description of Pope's visit to Bombay in John W. O'Malley, *What Happened at Vatican II* (Cambridge, MA: Harvard University Press, 2010), 247–48.

276 **the "utter simplicity"**: Description of Pope's visit to Bombay in O'Malley, *What Happened at Vatican II*.

276 **sixty-seven hours in India**: Letter from Lawrencetta Veeneman to her family, December 17, 1964.

276 **"Would that the nations"**: Text of Pope's address to non-Christians in Bombay, *New York Times*, December 4, 1964; "Paul to India," *New York Times*, December 6, 1964.

276 **"the missionary pope"**: "Paul to India," *New York Times*.

277 **"Yes, the Pope is becoming a missionary"**: "Paul to India," *New York Times*.

277 **forty-five dollars for two hundred pictures**: Letter from Lawrencetta Veeneman to her family, June 10, 1965.

277 **Mary Martha had arrived**: Interview with Margaret Thornton, 2017; letter from Lawrencetta Veeneman to her family, September 14, 1964.

277 Dr. Wiss stayed in New York: Interview with Margaret Thornton, 2017.

278 Mary Martha spent some time: Interview with Margaret Thornton, 2017.

278 she called useless bureaucrats: Interview with John Wiss, August 8, 2017.

278 "A few more months": Letter from Lawrencetta Veeneman to her family, December 17, 1964, and January 8, 1965.

278 Jack Wiss died: Annals of the Mokameh Mission, February 8, 1964; John Wiss obituary.

279 It began with a letter: Letter from Reverend Thomas Noa, bishop of Marquette, Michigan, to Mother Lucille, July 16, 1965; biographical records from Sisters of Charity of Nazareth Archival Center.

279 Mother Lucille wrote to the Vatican: Letter from Mother Lucille to Sacred Congregation for the Affairs of the Religious, July 20, 1965; biographical records from Sisters of Charity of Nazareth Archival Center.

280 "asking for a dispensation": Letter from Archdiocese of Louisville to Mother General, August 25, 1965; biographical records from Sisters of Charity of Nazareth Archival Center.

280 spent the summer together: Interviews with Margaret Thornton, 2017.

280 They spent the summer: Interviews with Margaret Thornton, 2017.

281 Frontier Nursing Service: Letter from Helen Browne to Sister Margaret Vincent, August 2, 1965;. biographical records from Sisters of Charity of Nazareth Archival Center.

281 except for one incident: Interviews with Margaret Thornton, 2017.

281 Dr. Pauline Fox: Interview with Dr. Pauline Fox, March 2017.

282 raising orchids in the garden: Interview with Dr. Pauline Fox, March 2017; Mary Martha Wiss obituary.

282 share of memorable cases: Interview with Dr. Pauline Fox, March 2017.

282 two of the last Vatican II documents: O'Malley, *What Happened at Vatican II*, 319.

283 pages worth of translated excerpts: "Sharing of Supreme Churchly Power by the Pontiff and the Bishops Is Proclaimed," *New York Times*, October 29, 1965.

284 Anne Elizabeth to Bangalore: Annals of the Mokameh Mission, March 31, June 21, and July 1, 1965; saying Mass in Hindi, letter from Lawrencetta Veeneman to her family, January 8, 1965.

284 Leela went with a group: Interview with Leela Thomas, March 2016.

284 Elizabeth briefly went back: Interview with Elizabeth, March 2016.

284 Celine found a different path: Interview with Celine Minj, January 2018.

285 Lawrencetta made a trip: Letter from Lawrencetta Veeneman to her family, April 2, 1965.

285 Johnson helicoptered to Liberty Island: President Lyndon B. Johnson's Remarks at the Signing of the Immigration Bill Liberty Island, New York, October 3, 1965, https://www.youtube.com/watch?v=oQNP5XKMNls.

285 deliver a speech at the foot: President Lyndon B. Johnson's Remarks at the Signing of the Immigration Bill Liberty Island, text online at LBJ Presidential Library, http://www.lbjlibrary.org/lyndon-baines-johnson/timeline/lbj-on-immigration.

285 Johnson was riding the momentum: Anna Diamond, "The 1924 Law That Slammed the Door on Immigrants and the Politicians Who Pushed It Back Open," *Smithsonian Magazine*, May 19, 2020, https://www.smithsonianmag.com/history/1924-law-slammed-door-immigrants-and-politicians-who-pushed-it-back-open-180974910/; from Diamond's interview with Jia Lynn Yang, author of *One Mighty and Irresistible Tide: The Epic Struggle Over American Immigration, 1924–1965* (New York: W. W. Norton & Company, 2020).

CONCLUSION

290 messages on social media: https://www.facebook.com/NazarethHospitalMokamaSCN.

EPILOGUE

295 died at the age of eighty-eight: Biographical records from Sisters of Charity of Nazareth Archival Center; interview with Father Dismas Veeneman, March 28, 2017.

295 died in Mokama in 2015: Biographical records from Sisters of Charity of Nazareth Archival Center; Spalding Hurst, "Ann Roberta Powers, SCN—A Mystical Missionary Leaves Behind Her Legacy in India," June 29, 2015, Sisters of Charity of Nazareth website, https://scnfamily.org/ann-roberta-powers-scn-a-mystical-missionary-leaves-behind-her-legacy-in-india/comment-page-1/.

295 He went to the United States: Patricia Kelley, *Fifty Monsoons: Ministry of Change Through Women of India* (New York: Harmony House Publishers, 1999), 108; letter from Lawrencetta Veeneman to her family, June 7, 1960; letter from Mary Martha Wiss to her family, June 12, 1960.

296 Dan Rice became close: Kelley, *Fifty Monsoons*, 247–49.

296 Jim Cox wrote a history: Kelley, *Fifty Monsoons*, 141; Jim Cox, *We Band of Brothers: Sketches of Patna Jesuits* (India: Patna Jesuit Society, 1994).

296 Dolores Greenwell, the young sister: Spalding Hurst, "Sister Dolores Greenwell, SCN," August 21, 2015, of Sisters of Charity of Nazareth website, https://scnfamily.org/sister_dolores/.

296 as he was preparing to go to Mass: Detailed account of his death and burial at Mokama in letter from Lawrencetta Veeneman to her family, August 8, 1965; also in Annals of the Mokameh Mission, July 20, 1965.

296 had three children: Babs Gillard obituary; Eric Lazaro obituary.

296 Sister Charles Miriam Holt reverted: Biographical records from Sisters of Charity of Nazareth Archival Center; letter from Lawrencetta Veeneman to her family, May 8, 1961.

297 left India in 1962: Biographical records from Sisters of Charity of Nazareth Archival Center; permanent departure of Crescentia, letter from Lawrencetta Veeneman to her family, May 31, 1962.

297 Sister Florence Joseph Sauer: Biographical records from Sisters of Charity of Nazareth Archival Center.

297 Sister Ann Cornelius Curran: Biographical records from Sisters of Charity of Nazareth Archival Center; biography from Sisters of St. Joseph the Worker.

298 Dr. Wiss moved with Dr. Fox: Interview with Dr. Pauline Fox, 2017; Mary Wiss obituary.

298 Celine Minj had a long career: Interview with Celine Minj, 2018.

298 Sister Bridget Kappalumakal: Kelley, *Fifty Monsoons*, 412.

298 Leela Thomas moved to Canada: Interview with Leela Thomas, April 2016.

Bibliography

"11 Killed, 72 Hurt in Calcutta Riots." Associated Press. *New York Times*, October 28, 1946.

"130 Ordained as Priests in Colorful Bombay Rites." *The Voice*, December 11, 1964.

"3600 Children at Rally Receive Communion." *The Voice*, December 11, 1964.

"15,000-Sq.-Mile Area Floods in Bihar." *Times of India*, October 7, 1961.

American Journal of Nursing 44, no. 10 (October 1944): 994–1010.

"The Battered Face of Bihar." *Times of India*, October 22, 1961.

"Big Increase in Food Is Planned for India." *New York Times*, May 23, 1948.

"Bihar Dead Put at 1,000." *New York Times*, October 10, 1961.

"Bihar Floods Exact Toll of Nearly 900 Human Lives." *Times of India*, October 10, 1961.

"Flood Toll in Bihar Has Risen to 908." *Times of India*, October 11, 1961.

"Four-Day Deluge Ends." *Times of India* News Service, October 5, 1961.

"Hundreds Killed in Bihar Floods." *Times of India*, October 8, 1961.

"Nehru May Survey Flood Damage." *Times of India*, October 11, 1961.

"Paul to India." *New York Times*, December 6, 1964.

"Peace Picture on Home Front Summarized." (Louisville) *Courier-Journal*, August 13, 1945.

"Peace Sends Volcano of Riotous Joy Pouring Down Fourth Street." (Louisville) *Courier-Journal*, August 15, 1945.

"Pope Paul Flies to Rites in India." *New York Times*, December 2, 1964.

"S Is for Sister and also Surgeon." *Ohio State University Monthly*, November 1959.

"Sharing of Supreme Churchly Power by the Pontiff and the Bishops Is Proclaimed." *New York Times*, October 29, 1965.

Arnow, Harriette Louisa Simpson. *The Collected Short Stories of Harriette Simpson Arnow*. East Lansing, MI: University of Michigan Press, 2005.

Bayly, Christopher, and Tim Harper. *Forgotten Armies: The Fall of British Asia 1941–45*. Cambridge, MA: Belknap Press of Harvard University Press, 2005.

Bingham, Sallie. *The Blue Box: Three Lives in Letters*. Louisville: Sarabande Books, 2014.

———. *Passion and Prejudice: A Family Memoir*. New York: Alfred A. Knopf, 1989.

Bourke-White, Margaret. *Halfway to Freedom: A Report on the New India*. New York: Simon and Schuster, 1949.

Bowles, Chester. *A View from New Delhi: Selected Speeches and Writings, 1963–1969*. New Haven, CT: Yale University Press, 1969.

Brady, Thomas F. "Cardinal Opens Bombay Congress: 100,000 People Assemble for Eucharistic Session." *New York Times*, November 29, 1964.

Brannan, Beverly W., and David Horvath, eds. *A Kentucky Album: Farm Security Administration Photographs: 1935–1943*. Lexington, KY: University Press of Kentucky, 1986.

Brocato, Maria Vincent, and Mary Ellen Doyle. *Impelled by the Love of Christ: Sisters of Charity of Nazareth Kentucky, 1948–1960*. Nazareth, KY: Sisters of Charity of Nazareth, 2012.

Burton, Katherine. *According to the Pattern: The Story of Dr Agnes McLaren and the Society of Catholic Medical Missionaries*. New York: Longmans Green & Co, 1946.

Butalia, Urvashi. *The Other Side of Silence: Voices from the Partition of India*. New Delhi, India: Penguin Books India, 1998.

Caudill, Harry M. *Night Comes to the Cumberlands: A Biography of a Depressed Area*. Boston: Little, Brown, 1963.

Chaudhuri, Nirad C. *Thy Hand Great Anarch! India 1921–1952*. Boston: Addison-Wesley, 1989.

Damodaran, Vinita. *Broken Promises: Popular Protest, Indian Nationalism and the Congress Party in Bihar, 1935–1946*. Delhi, New York: Oxford University Press, 1992.

Datta, K. K. *History of the Freedom Movement in Bihar*. Patna: Government of Bihar, 1958.

Diamond, Anna. "The 1924 Law That Slammed the Door on Immigrants and the Politicians Who Pushed It Back Open," *Smithsonian Magazine*, May 19, 2020.

Doyle, Mary Ellen. *Pioneer Spirit: Catherine Spalding, Sister of Charity of Nazareth*. Lexington: University Press of Kentucky, 2006.

Dries, Angelyn, "'Fire and Flame': Anna Dengel and the Medical Mission to Women and Children." *Missiology*, 2016.

———. *The Missionary Movement in American Catholic History*. Maryknoll, NY: Orbis Books, 1998.

Dudziak, Mary L. *Cold War Civil Rights: Race and the Image of American Democracy*. Princeton, NJ: Princeton University Press, 2000.

Ebright, Donald F. *Free India: The First Five Years. An Account of the 1947 Riots, Refugees, Relief and Rehabilitation*. Nashville, TN: Parthenon Press, 1954.

Elgin, Kathleen. *Nun: A Gallery of Sisters*. New York: Random House, 1964.

Fay, Peter Ward. *The Forgotten Army: India's Armed Struggle for Independence 1942–45*. Ann Arbor: University of Michigan Press, 1993.

FitzGerald, David S., and David Cook-Martín. "The Geopolitical Origins of the U.S. Immigration Act of 1965." In *Culling the Masses· The Democratic Origins of Racist Immigration Policy in the Americas*. Cambridge, MA: Harvard University Press, 2014.

Galbraith, John Kenneth. *Ambassador's Journal: A Personal Account of the Kennedy Years*. New York: Houghton Mifflin, 1969.

Gish, Shirley. *Country Doctor: The Story of Dr. Claire Louise Caudill*. Lexington, KY: University Press of Kentucky, 1999.

Gopalan, A. K. *Kerala Past and Present*. London: Lawrence & Wishart, 1959.

Guha, Ramachandra. *Gandhi: The Years that Changed the World, 1914–1948*. New York: Alfred A. Knopf, 2018.

———. *India After Gandhi: The History of the World's Largest Democracy*. New York: HarperCollins, 2007.

Hajari, Nisid. *Midnight's Furies: The Deadly Legacy of India's Partition.* New York: Houghton Mifflin Harcourt, 2015.

Halperin, Rhoda. *The Livelihood of Kin: Making Ends Meet "The Kentucky Way."* Austin: University of Texas Press, 1990.

Hess, Gary R. *America Encounters India, 1941–47.* Baltimore, MD: Johns Hopkins Press, 1971.

Holl, Richard E. *Committed to Victory: The Kentucky Home Front During World War II.* Lexington: University Press of Kentucky, 2015.

Irvin, Helen Deiss. *Women in Kentucky.* Lexington: University Press of Kentucky, 1979.

Jackson, Kathi. *They Called Them Angels: American Military Nurses of World War II.* Westport, CT: Praeger, 2000.

Jhabvala, Ruth Prawer. *The Nature of Passion: A Novel.* New York: W. W. Norton, 1957.

Kalapura, Jose, ed. *Christian Missions in Bihar and Jharkhand Till 1947: A Study by P. C. Horo.* New Delhi: Christian World Imprints, 2014.

Karaka, D. F. *Betrayal in India.* London: Victor Gollancz, 1950.

———. *I've Shed My Tears: A Candid View of Resurgent India.* New York: D. Appleton-Century, 1947.

Karnad, Raghu. *Farthest Field: An Indian Story of the Second World War.* New York: W. W. Norton, 2015.

Karsell, Tom. "First Sister of Charity to Become Physician Completes Four-Year Residency in Surgery." (Louisville) *Courier-Journal*, July 5, 1958.

Kelley, Patricia. *Fifty Monsoons: Ministry of Change Through Women of India.* New York: Harmony House Publishers, 1999.

Kelley, Patricia, Elaine McCarron, and Rachel Willett. *Impelled by the Love of Christ: Sisters of Charity of Nazareth Kentucky, 1936–1948.* Nazareth, KY: Sisters of Charity of Nazareth, 2013.

Kerala State, Bureau of Economics and Statistics. *Women in Kerala.* Trivandrum: Government of Kerala, 1978.

Khan, Yasmin. *The Great Partition: The Making of India and Pakistan.* New Haven, CT: Yale University Press, 2007.

———. *The Raj at War: A People's History of India's Second World War.* Random House India, 2015.

Kochendoerfer, Violet A. *One Woman's World War II*. Lexington: University Press of Kentucky, 1994.

McGill, Anna Blanche. *The Sisters of Charity of Nazareth Kentucky*. New York: Encyclopedia Press, 1917.

Maes, Camillus Paul. *The Life of Rev. Charles Nerinckx: With a Chapter on the Early Catholic Missions of Kentucky; Copious Notes on the Progress of Catholicity in the United States of America, from 1800 to 1825; an Account of the Establishment of the Society of Jesus in Missouri; and an Historical Sketch of the Sisterhood of Loretto in Kentucky, Missouri, New Mexico, Etc.* Cincinnati, OH: R. Clarke & Company, 1880.

Mansergh, Nicholas, ed. *The Transfer of Power 1942–47.* Volume I, Cripps Mission; Volume II, Quit India; Volume III, Reassertion of Authority. London: Her Majesty's Stationery Office, 1971.

Marston, Daniel. *The Indian Army and the End of the Raj: Decolonising the Subcontinent*. Cambridge: Cambridge University Press, 2014.

Mason, Bobbie Ann. *Clear Springs*. New York: Random House, 1999.

Mathew, K. M. *Annamma: Mrs. K. M. Mathew: A Book of Memories*. New Delhi: Penguin Books India, 2005.

McConkey, James. *Rowan's Progress*. New York: Pantheon Books, 1992.

McEuen, Melissa, and Thomas H. Appleton, Jr. *Kentucky Women: Their Lives and Times*. Athens and London: University of Georgia Press.

Mehta, Ved. *Walking the Indian Streets*. Boston: Little, Brown and Company, 1959.

Montell, William Lynwood. *Tales from Kentucky Doctors*. Ukraine: University Press of Kentucky, 2008.

Moon, Penderel. *Divide and Quit: An Eyewitness Account of the Partition of India*. London: Chatto and Windus, 1961.

Muething, Sister Eugenia. *Nazareth Along the Banks of the Ganges, 1947–1990*. New York: Harmony House Publishers, 1997.

Mukerjee, Madhusree. *Churchill's Secret War: The British Empire and the Ravaging of India During World War II*. New York: Basic Books, 2010.

Nayaran, Badri. *Documenting Dissent: Contesting Fables, Contested Minorities and Dalit Political Discourse*. Shimla: Indian Institute of Advanced Study, 2001.

Pandey, Gyanendra. "The Revolt of August 1942 in Eastern UP and Bihar." In *The Indian Nation in 1942*. Edited by Gyanendra Pandey. Calcutta: Center for Studies in Social Sciences, 1988.

Poole, Ernest. *Nurses on Horseback*. New York: Macmillan Company, 1932.

Powers, Sister Ann Roberta, SCN. "My Story." Sisters of Charity of Nazareth Archival Center, July 2005.

Raghavan, Srinath. *India's War: World War II and the Making of Modern South Asia*. New York: Basic Books, 2016.

Report of the Health Survey and Development Committee, Vols. 1, 2, and 3. Calcutta: Government of India Press, 1946.

Ridge, Mian. "Fadeout for a Culture That's Neither Indian Nor British," *New York Times*, August 14, 2010.

Roland, Charles P. *The Improbable Era: The South Since World War II*. Lexington: University Press of Kentucky, 1975.

Rynne, Xavier. "Letter from Vatican City," *New Yorker*, December 25, 1965.

Shousha, Aly Tewfik. "Cholera Epidemic in Egypt (1947)," *Bulletin of the World Health Organization 1*, no. 2 (1948): 353–81.

Spillane, James Maria. *Kentucky Spring*. St. Meinrad, IN: Abbey Press, 1968.

———. *Summer Winds: Sisters of Charity of Nazareth Kentucky 1859–1912*. St. Meinrad, IN: Abbey Press, 1991.

Thomas, Sonja. *Privileged Minorities: Syrian Christianity, Gender, and Minority Rights in Postcolonial India*. Seattle: University of Washington Press, 2018.

Tomblin, Barbara Brooks. *G.I. Nightingales: The Army Nurse Corps in World War II*. Lexington: University Press of Kentucky, 1996.

Tuker, Francis. *While Memory Serves*. London: Cassell, 1950.

Tyler, Bruce. *Louisville in World War II*. Charleston, SC: Arcadia Publishing, 2005.

Vaishnav, Milan. *When Crime Pays: Money and Muscle in Indian Politics*. New Haven, CT: Yale University Press, 2017.

Whitehead, Andrew. "India: A People Partitioned," Oral Archive, BBC World Service, 1997.

Zachariah, Benjamin. *Ideas of Developing India: An Intellectual and Social History, 1930–1950*. Oxford: Oxford University Press, 2005.